All I Want For Christm

By Grace Winter

Copyright
©Grace Winter 2008

Dedication

For my children; the love, inspiration and blessing that your existence has given to me.

For Jude; a remarkable mother, teacher, writer and friend. Thank you for always being there and giving so much no matter how much hard work I have been.

For the couples who kindly shared their stories with me in the hope it will inspire and answer questions for others.

Preface

When I had to try IVF (In Vitro Fertilization) I had no idea of the effects it would have on me, my marriage, my family and friends. Neither had any of the other IVF couples I'd met. If there had been a book out there with the unique approach of the male and female perspective, focusing on emotions and relationships as opposed to the technicalities, we'd all have purchased it. So here it is. More importantly, this is not just aimed at couples facing or having gone through IVF but at their family and friends to offer help with maintaining relationships.

It's not a textbook about IVF treatment. It's about people and the journey prior, during and after IVF. It covers pregnancy, strained relationships in all areas, divorce, support, donors, isolation, depression, elation, love, miracles and a whole lot more. All the case studies are real. People have opened up and shared their unique experience and I have changed names in the book, including my own, to preserve confidentiality, so that we can open up for you, the reader, in the hope that our experiences will help you with your unanswered questions, emotions and relationships.

I have added humour and lightness where possible to lift the mood of the topic. It should answer all the questions parents, siblings, men and women are unable to ask and which no other book currently on the market addresses. It approaches IVF differently, showing that it is more than just about becoming a parent. It is inspirational, informative and gripping.

This is a powerful subject covering the stories of seven couples and their infertility. Unlike other books currently on the market it covers the journey of infertility, IVF and the early years with children. It is my own experience wrapped around six other couples short stories, uniquely offering both the male and female perspective, helping a variety of people to understand what such couples have to face. Chapters are clearly titled for easy reading and are based upon our memories, diaries and experiences and should not be used as factual with regards to IVF procedures which are always changing – always consult a professional for up to date advice. We apologise to anyone we may offend or upset with our stories and have written this to help people and not to deliberately offend anyone.

Prologue

I'm feeling fearful on far too many levels today. The most immediate fear is the vast amount of cows grazing in the overgrown field around me - I'm terrified of cows - of being one of the fifteen unlucky souls killed by one each year while walking a dog. I prefer to switch off and walk in a world of my own without having to keep a nervous eye on the herd. I'm watching my puppy, Fudge, a fox red Labrador Retriever, thrilled to be catching the scent of pheasants and deer. I envy her freedom to enjoy life. Her mind is not tormented by unachieved goals, past baggage, sleep deprivation, depression, resentment, anger – ferocious anger, fear, worry.

She lives in the moment, something I haven't been able to do in a long time. She's three months old and has no thoughts about her future; whether or not I'll give her the opportunity to become a mother one day, or indeed sort that out for herself, or where her life will lead. I wish I could be like that. I was thirty four and terrified of my age and the fact that each year jeopardised yet another chance of me bearing a child. I was considered young in the world of IVF and yet motherhood-out-of-reach made me feel ancient. I worked in Information Technology, which was still very male dominated, and had never felt oppressed or resentful towards men until now: the fact that they had no age limit on procreation or felt the tick-tock of the clock ate away at me with a vengeance. I was not the sort of woman to cope with never having children: it was not something I felt I could get through. It meant everything to me. EVERYTHING. Life would be utterly pointless otherwise.

The Thames is beautiful today; tranquil and sunny. A heron haunts his usual place, ducks and swans glide along lazily until Fudge jumps in and disturbs them - she's having so much fun. I've often looked into this water with melancholy and despair, considering drowning and ending it all. This is where infertility took me: the frustration of not having anything to fix and facing the heartbreak of failure month after month. Almost five years. Fifty six months. Two hundred and forty three weeks. Devastating. Some months turned me insane, as if my head was completely damaged with all the scary negative thoughts, unable to think outside of the dark dreary fog. What was wrong with me? I was vividly aware that I was mentally and physically damaged.

Today is different. Melancholy has no current hold over me and suicidal thoughts are far from my mind. I have hope. Yesterday was a colossal day at the hospital and I could be carrying life. It was December 6th and all I wanted for Christmas was a baby.

Table of Contents

Contents

Dedication 3

Preface 4

Prologue 6

Table of Contents 8

Chapter 1 - Crushing Broodiness 9

Chapter 2 – The Dark Dingy Road Of Relentless Failing IVF 29

Chapter 3 – Darren and Julie 43

Chapter 4 - Divine Pregnancy: Here they come 53

Chapter 5 - Stephen and Claire 75

Chapter 6 - The Art Of Blundering Breastfeeding 87

Chapter 7 – Adam and Kelly 102

Chapter 8 - The Magnanimous First Year 110

Chapter 9 – Mark and Susan 129

Chapter 10 - Callously Deserted 144

Chapter 11 - Michael and Fiona 160

Chapter 12 - Unfettered Life As A Single Mum 166

Chapter 13 – Cliff and Jane 181

Chapter 14 - Exultation For A Fresh Start 194

Chapter 1 - Crushing Broodiness

I could hear my son waking up and calling out to me but I was too tired to get up. My eyes felt glued together and refused to open and my body was numb. I heard him climb out of bed – wasn't he in a cot? – and toddle into my room. He's trying to climb up onto the bed - I'm unable to move or help. He just about manages it and snuggles into me. I kiss his forehead and run my fingers through his thick curly brown hair – so wavy and luscious. Finally, I open my eyes just enough to see his bright blue eyes smiling down on me.

"Hey baby," I whisper, kissing him on his little button nose before reaching for the television controls.

"Hey, honey," James murmurs, half asleep, assuming I was talking to him and snuggles closer into my back. I smile, turn on some cartoons, breathe in my sons smell and drift back into sleep.

I awake with a start, very aware of the silence in the room and the undeniable fact that my toddler was missing. Perhaps James had taken him downstairs so I could have a lie in? But as I turned over I could feel James lying asleep beside me. I sit bolt upright. Something was wrong – where had he gone? I scan the room. Had I closed the stair gate? Please God, don't let him have fallen down the stairs! Just a minute, what happened to the cartoons? The television was off, the controls were on the windowsill – how had they gotten over there? James was fast asleep and my son had gone!

"Where is he?" I screech hysterically, patting the duvet in futile hope.

"Who?" James asked, rubbing his eyes and looking up at my frantic face.

"He was here, he was watching—" the words catch in my throat and I feel my blood run cold.

James watches the expressions pass over my face, knowing what was coming, helpless to do anything to help, as I fully awoke and reality sank in: I didn't have a son. It had all been a horrifying dream – that awful recurring dream that haunts me relentlessly.

"Did you have another one of those dreams?" he asked, turning to cuddle me.

I nod and burst into tears, sobbing into his chest. He strokes my hair, feeling my pain and wishing desperately that he could do something, anything, to stop it.

"It was so real – I can still see his little face – perfectly – I know exactly what he looks like. Why can I still smell him!"

"It's going to be OK, Grace, I promise," he said but it was an empty promise – how could he know?

And then, just to rub insult into injury, the pains began in my lower back – the sort that meant only one thing. In order to not worry James further, I sluggishly got out of bed, shoulders slumped, and went to the bathroom. I had, as I guessed, started my period. Another unwanted period. I was devastated. I sobbed as I showered and desperately tried to keep the noise down but no doubt he knew what I was up to. It must have been horrible lying helplessly in bed hearing me. I felt guilty for not being able to hold myself together – shouldn't I be able to cope with this by now? Why is each month as bad as the first? I felt as if I was going crazy – my mind was out of control – and nothing mattered but this limbo of infertility and needing to get out of it. I couldn't focus on work, friends, family, life – nothing but this black existence. I was trapped in it and there was only one way out – to get pregnant.

If you desperately want children and are hell-bent on achieving that then there is no switching off or turning back. It's not like saying you would like a dog, a boat, a holiday. It becomes mental and physical, your entire body and mindset alters. There is a yearning that cannot be ignored, consuming you entirely. Perhaps, with enough failure or difficulty, you can come to terms with it but there is still something wrong – or missing. With time this also may be overcome – for some. For others, it will remain a lifelong curse, regret, hole, bitterness or sadness. Some fill the gap with adopting horses, or other animals, children, elderly or disabled people in need. Some fill the gaping hole with material objects that are never enough. The bottom line, no matter how an individual handles it, is that it changes you for life from that moment on. Everything is different. It amazes me that one woman can feel such a desperate craving while another goes through life never feeling the need to have a child. For some, it can be as bad as losing a child because in a way you have lost a child – the one you so desperately craved. Rape, death, murder are the only things extreme enough to compete with the inability to have children in my experience. I had been raped and can honestly say that was easier to come to terms with than infertility – for me. Upon returning to the bedroom, I turn my red-rimmed eyes to James and take a shaky breath.

"Now we have to do it," I sadly announce.

He nodded.

This was my final defeat – it was time to face IVF.

***

We were referred to the same consultant that we had seen two years previously. I had not been ready to face it then, being thirty-two, and was determined to conceive naturally. They had tested James's sperm back then so we knew he had a fluctuating sperm count, which was very common, and that alone shouldn't prevent us getting pregnant in the long run. It was enough to qualify us for IVF. First, they would have to run tests on me and eliminate any problems on my side before we proceeded. Previously, I had not been ready for the intrusive tests. I still wasn't but the time had come to face the music. The tests took place remarkably fast and I received the results within six weeks. My ultrasound scan, to check my ovaries and womb, showed no problems and was horribly intrusive: I felt all my dignity had gone – smear tests paled in comparison. I learned that as far as intrusive goes, this was nothing compared to what was coming.

My blood tests were fine and I had no awful diseases. James had a semen test done and it wasn't great. They scheduled him in for another one in a few weeks time, explaining it was normal for the first one to show a low sperm count, and they would not form an opinion on just one sample because it varied so much over time. I was amazed, and jealous, to learn that a man produced new sperm approximately every three months whereas a woman created her lifelong batch of eggs before she was even born and could run out at anytime. Why couldn't we recreate more eggs later in life as and when needed? If a man could do it, why couldn't we? Why were we only able to create one batch of eggs while we were in the womb? It didn't make sense to me and I wondered if all mammals were the same or whether it's was human thing? It certainly seemed unfair.

They scheduled me in for a Laparoscopy and dye. I would not be conscious for it. I was so nervous as they dressed me in the hospital gown and injected me with the anaesthetic. I had never spent any time in hospital and it was all new and scary. I felt vulnerable and resented having to go through this. All I kept thinking was how easy James had got it – if only all I had to do was come in a cup! Instead, I was being shaved, stripped, prodded, poked – all I wanted was a sexy night of passion followed by a happy declaration that something beautiful was created in the process. The anaesthetist was lovely and even rubbed some cream on my hand so I couldn't feel the needle go in – he could tell how nervous I was and kept me distracted with all sorts of information about himself – it was very interesting at the time but I instantly forgot the conversation. A Laparoscopy involved a small incision near the navel and a laparoscope (a small telescope) was inserted to allow inspection of the womb and fallopian tubes. They checked the fallopian tubes and pelvic area, looked for scar tissue and endometriosis; which I had a small amount of but not enough to cause infertility or pay any attention to. A dye was injected through the cervix to see if it ran through the fallopian tubes – checking for blockages. There was nothing wrong anywhere. James showed a better sperm count on his second test and we were again told that it shouldn't affect us getting pregnant in the long term because it wasn't always low and so there was no main reason we couldn't get pregnant naturally.

"You could keep trying," the consultant said, as I listened, stunned.

I just wanted there to be an exact cause so that we could correct it – this got us nowhere.

"Or, you can try for another year and then next year, when you reach the age of thirty-five, you will be entitled to a round of IVF on the NHS."

"Can't we have that now?" James asked.

"No, Grace has to be thirty-five to qualify."

"But then another year has passed, I'm that bit older and the odds get less favourable," I whispered.

"Yes, this is true," the consultant said. "Many couples opt to pay for IVF now, having age on their side, but you won't get any on the NHS then. It's up to you. You certainly qualify for IVF but you would have to pay privately and it isn't cheap. You need to think about it and decide what you want to do."

"We've wasted enough time and have savings so let's go for it," I say, anxiously.

"Do you both want to discuss it first?"

"No," I said firmly.

"We've already discussed it and we knew this might happen. We're happy to go ahead," James explained.

"OK, I'll schedule you in for the IVF presentation evening and start the process, it will take a few weeks," he told us.

"Can we wait about six months?" I asked.

"Yes, but then why not wait a year and get it done on the NHS?"

"Because I want us to have the extra time to eat even more healthily, build up a new batch of sperm and do at least three months of acupuncture," I explained, somewhat robotically, remembering the list of things that I had read with the intention of incorporating absolutely everything into our even healthier than normal life style. "But I'm also conscious of time and want as many months on my side as possible."

"That's not a problem; the presentation will explain everything to you."

"There's really nothing wrong?" I had become convinced that I had Chlamydia or problem ovaries or no eggs.

"No, Grace, there is nothing wrong. Most couples going through IVF have no obvious reason as to why they need to have it. We could do further tests and try to identify the actual cause, if there is any, but it isn't worth the time and cost and will still result in IVF. The presentation will cover all the options available to you."

"Thanks for your time," James said, getting up and pulling my numb body with him.

"Oh, and James?" the consultant said.

"Yes?"

"Stop cycling for the duration, it's not doing you any favours and is known to damage sperm."

James, never one for words, merely nodded.

I felt sick. Disappointed. Terrified. I felt worthless. There was no warmth or understanding from the consultant; this was merely another day on the same old job and our emotions seemed irrelevant.

***

I did what I do with any project – went full throttle and immersed myself into achieving it with total commitment. I learned all there was to know, read and listened to everyone's stories, took on board every little thing that could help or could hinder and adopted it into my lifestyle and made James do the same. I immediately scheduled us both in for acupuncture, cut out dairy, made James swallow the vilest of vegetable and fruit smoothies: the expression on his face as he gulped down the darkest green cabbage, spinach, courgette, carrot and red pepper smoothie always made me laugh. He would give me the dirtiest of looks as he swallowed and retched until it had all gone. He could do over dramatic rather well. We did every possible thing every book in the world told us to do. I was focused; obsessed; possessed. James almost played ball. In one way, he was really supportive and in another he seemed to be doing everything the consultant had told him not to – cycling, running his bath far too hot so that even I couldn't get in it over half an hour later and drinking far too much alcohol. I watched him, like a hawk, with narrowed eyes.

Our lives were put on hold as we waited the few weeks until the presentation. I painfully monitored my periods, as usual, and we still attempted to get pregnant naturally – I couldn't give up hope. I didn't want to do IVF. However, I had committed to it now and had to change my mind-set and be more positive than I had ever been in my entire life. I got chickens – because one book told me they were a sign of fertility and having such fertile animals around helped your body clock change – so in came two pet chickens. I got a puppy – Fudge. I quit work since I was lucky enough to be in a position to do so, being self employed, and would probably end up losing a contract anyway, if not for being unprofessionally emotional then for being pregnant – as was often the way in my line of business. I had hired and fired, or tried to hire, enough to know what was really acceptable and cringed many times when people were deliberately not hired, or let go, for being too old, likely to need maternity leave or were already pregnant. As soon as anyone found out I was a pregnant IT Contractor they would terminate my contract. IT was still a young man's world and work where this was not the case was very hard to find, especially at my managerial level. I'd seen how it worked and I at didn't want the indignity of being let go that way so I chose to do it myself. In addition, contracts were currently few and far between and competition was high. The odds were against me. I had savings

To pass the time I doted on Fudge, which temporarily fulfilled my nurturing need, I volunteered at a junior school teaching excel after class because, apparently, being around children helped too. I did everything from the small to the extreme in order to optimise my chances of success. I focused on nothing more than that and told myself we would only have to do it once – mind over matter was all I believed in. James and I had an argument, a big one, because he had signed up to do the Tourmalet cycle ride in Spain that July. He had never done it before and had just been told not to cycle. I was furious. James went to bed in a strop and I got too drunk on my own downstairs while moaning to my friends on the phone. A close friend of mine suggested that he didn't seem as if he wanted children and was it me pushing him into it? I began to wonder if this was the case since he had signed up to so much cycling. James denied it, insisted that he did want children and that he just didn't believe the consultant about cycling.

"I read online that it doesn't affect your sperm at all," he argued.

"You can always find two arguments for every subject, especially online, but the idea is we follow the advice of the consultant for the next six months – this is it – this is show time!" I yelled.

"It won't make any difference," he said stubbornly.

"You don't really want children! All you want is to keep me in a little bubble all to yourself – you've scared off my family, you've scared off most of my friends and they all call you a feeder because you've made me fat and just want me all to yourself," it was a slight exaggeration said in anger.

"Don't be stupid! You're family is twisted."

"So are yours!"

"Yes, but not as much as yours!"

"Oh God, listen to us, now we're arguing over whose family is worse," I started to cry.

"I'm sick of this!" he walked away.

I sobbed on the floor and drank some more and called some more friends. I couldn't believe he was doing this, not now! As he boasted about it to his friends, yet hardly did any proper training, I wondered if this was his way of boosting his confidence because of his sperm count. However, it went completely against our IVF goal and I couldn't understand it. I hated him. I had dated a triathalete once and knew the sort of training required for such an event – he wasn't doing it – he wasn't focused. I just didn't understand what he was up to – it seemed as if he was just doing it to spite me rather than wanting to do it for himself. Or perhaps he wanted to restrict the training because he felt guilty cycling even though he had signed up for it. It was simply nonsensical. I watched him, wondering what on earth was going on, and supported him on the surface. I went to France with him, drove him everywhere, talked about nothing but him and his cycling, dropped him off in the pouring rain at four in the morning, raced to each point in my car to stand, cheer, clap, and shout "I love you" as loud as I could and look the supportive wife. Deep down I hated him for doing this because I couldn't understand it. IVF was now four months away – barely enough time for him to create another batch of fresh sperm after he had squished and killed them all on this bike ride.

As it happened, he was out of the Tourmalet in the first two hours because he wasn't fast enough and didn't get to the checkpoint on time. He was 12 minutes over the time limit. He was furious, arguing with them, blaming them but there was nothing he could do and they were used to such arguments so ignored him until he gave up. The rules were simple: reach each check point within a given time or you are out. James was simply not fit enough for such an event. I was spitefully pleased he had failed, hoping for limited sperm damage, and then felt immediately guilty so took him out to lunch, got him drunk and held his hand as he went on about the unfairness of it all and how someone had cut him up, causing him to fall behind and he hadn't planned on it pouring down of rain. Well, it was a horrendous downpour and I had felt sorry for him soaked to the skin, cycling as fast as he could with his little cherry cheeks and frozen hands. He was a fair weather cyclist so the odds had been against him. My spite started to subside and my pity took over.

"I'm really sorry," I whispered, kissing his hand.

"I know. I promise I won't cycle anymore until IVF is over, OK?"

"OK."

He kept his promise.

***

The years of trying to conceive naturally had taken its toll on us. It was also one of the best forms of contraceptives. There was nothing like baby-making and having sex for a purpose to destroy your sex drive and passion. Of course, we didn't see this at first; it just crept up on us. I had always had a great sex drive and didn't think anything could kill it so stone dead – and no matter what we tried we couldn't get it back. Month by month our lives began to rotate around chore-like intercourse and periods. Nothing mattered but making a family. It consumed us in ways I never thought possible. The months became years and still the time passed. I stopped laughing and smiling. I became very serious and deeply miserable. I felt distant from every social gathering and felt far from normal. I came from a large family with more children than adults and had spent most of my life surrounded by children. I even worked as a nanny in the UK and abroad – children was all I cared about. I wrote a poem about one little girl in particular and had it published in a small magazine while I was in the States. To my good fortune, a decade later her parents flew with this girl over to the UK so that she could be a bridesmaid at my wedding. I felt honoured and lucky because I really loved this family.

I had been broody for as long as I could remember. My sister had been the same – she desperately wanted children from as young as eleven. She didn't wait as long as me and went on to have three children from age twenty. I wanted a career first. What the hell were we thinking? What stupid berk told us to focus on our career and have children later in life so that we could achieve everything? I did achieve the career, prior to finding someone to marry, hoping beyond hope that he wasn't going to be a prize bum and leave me as a single mother, or refuse to help, or sleep with a younger girl with tight boobs and a flat stomach. Our bodies were not in sync with our minds. We were ready to breed twenty years earlier.

My brain was not functioning as it used to and I became convinced that I was mentally damaged; deranged or insane on some level. I could not look at the world the way I used to and my mind was constantly invaded with negative and dark thoughts. I felt as if I lived on a different planet to everyone else. It took years to realise I was not alone and this was common – I could now understand how a woman gets to the point of being able to snatch another woman's baby – it messes up your head. I've met women who couldn't be in the same room as a baby or couldn't bear to talk about any of their friend's pregnancies and children. However, others were heartbroken when their friends concealed pregnancies and information from them, as I was. It was hard to guess the best way of handling women craving a child since there was no fixed rule: don't tell them and you might offend them; do tell them and it'll break their hearts. My decision with this dilemma was to try to treat women like me as normal as possible but don't go on about it too much – that's our problem to deal with – but leaving us out of the loop can be more painful than having to repeatedly listen to all the details. Ask what is preferred, if you value your friendship, and let them ask the questions.

I was the only person I knew personally who grabbed every baby and toddler that I could. I was that person at a party that took everyone's child and got him/her to sleep; a knack I had always had with young children, so that the parents could relax and enjoy themselves. I would sit or walk for hours holding their child and loving the warmth of it. I loved it when exhausted parents on flights looked as if they could take no more – in I stepped. Strangers accepted this since there was nowhere you could run off with their child on a plane. People in Europe do this for strangers all the time but we are so suspicious in this country that it's unheard of. I was a child-hogger and I couldn't get enough. I didn't have issues with this too often, people could tell I loved helping them out and appreciated it, whereas those who knew how desperately I wanted a baby gave me obvious pitiful glances and felt awkward. This would undoubtedly make me feel self-conscious and awkward too. Eventually, I only looked for such opportunities with people who didn't know my circumstances. If there was a party, wedding or any social event and a woman couldn't attend because her children were sick, I would be the one sitting in their hotel room helping them. I liked feeling part of their world, even with sick and grisly children, because it was where I most wanted to be. Drinking wine with everyone else felt empty, boring and pointless.

Young mothers often tell me they feel persecuted for having a child, aged nineteen or twenty, and I find it horrible that they are made to feel that way by so-called professionals. They ask if I think they are bad mothers or have lost any chance of a career. Absolutely not! She could fight for a career later on, much easier than fighting for a child. She was breeding precisely when nature intended her to, which is why it happened with that 'just one night'. Plus, they get funding and a crèche at university instead of their entire salary going directly onto childcare. Not like us, month after month, year after year, and still zilch. Mother Nature knew what she was doing. We did not. And yet, I believed older mothers have much to offer. We were more mature, grateful and financially stable. One of the biggest issues I had with my own parents was their immaturity – they were too young and had five children – they raised us as if they were our older siblings and not our parents. All they knew was how to bully, blackmail and control their children: gentle persuasive discipline was alien to them. Slippers, belts and table legs were normal punishment when guilt trips or blackmail failed. As with most debates, I think there were pro's and con's to being older or younger parents.

I was convinced that people on the Jeremy Kyle show would be better parents if they had to fight for those babies. Imagine what they could achieve if they put as much energy into parenting as they did into getting attention. My friend once cried when we watched the show: she has had miscarriage after miscarriage, was almost forty and sat listening to an ungrateful teenager arguing that getting totally drunk on mixed shots wasn't going to harm her baby at all, while her rundown parents pleaded with Jeremy Kyle to convince her otherwise. Why are they allowed to get pregnant and we weren't? Was it God's will? Why... Why... Why..!

If you want something bad enough you will go out there and get it. It never lands on your lap. No one owes you a thing. It was all up to you to serve yourself. I wanted children. James and I promised each other right from the start that we wouldn't blame each other and we tried hard to stick to that. We had seen friends split up over failing to conceive and we didn't want to be like them. We were certain that our relationship was better and stronger and that we had made this pact in good faith and truly believed we were achieving it. We were lying to ourselves. I blamed him: there was something wrong with him and it wasn't just his attitude. I tried to be understanding, I tried to be nice, but I was also starting to dislike him. The irony of it all ate away at my soul. I had wanted desperately to be a mother years before I met him. I picked a man who couldn't give me the only thing I could never compromise on. I felt truly ashamed of myself as a wife and as a woman for taking the easy way and blaming him. Outwardly, I appeared positive and encouraged him to take nutritional advice and follow the doctor's orders. Inside, I grieved that after all these years I picked a man who wasn't super fertile. I felt the bitterness eating at my heart and over the years I had turned nasty. Meanwhile, he also blamed me. When I couldn't cope I'd have an evening out drinking and smoking and would eat fast food – so off the scales of the routine we were supposed to be following - I became Mrs self-destructive. I hated myself so much, not only for the feeling that my body had let me down but because of the way I was treating the man of my dreams. He was also being self-destructive. We were not in good shape at all.

  I envisioned years of failed IVF, miscarriages, and heartache and wondered whether our relationship would sustain such an ordeal: it had already weakened by years of infertility and constant family dramas we desperately tried to avoid. We unplugged our phone more often than not; the abuse for not answering was the lesser evil. When we were strong, we worked well at handling our families. However, we were not working well together. James frequently instigated fights each month when I was ovulating making us occasionally miss the key times or, as I cringe to admit, going through with "the deed" with a bad taste in our mouths and under duress; it was horrible and left me wondering again if he actually wanted children. It was no way to live. He insisted that he did and couldn't understand why he acted the way he did either. It was confusing. During an argument, I made it clear that I had taken all I could stand and wanted to leave. I had always been clear that having children was the most important thing in my life. Upon mentioning the D-word he completely changed his attitude. He said we should stick together throughout three rounds of IVF and if it didn't work then we could separate if I still wanted to but he convinced me that there was nothing wrong with "us." I had his commitment – better late than never – and agreed to stay.

***

I was scared stiff of IVF – that was the bottom line. Just the idea of IVF was terrifying. I was quite the pragmatist and therefore the whole idea of being out of control, not having any real reason for years of fertility issues, and having to take this unknown, uncertain, and unguaranteed path was my idea of hell. No one can understand it, like so many other things in life, until they have experienced it. My brother and sister-in-law claimed they would only do it twice, and eight rounds later, thousands of pounds worse off, several trips to Spain for eggs, they were still persevering. When do you stop? At each round, you eliminate another problem which gives hope for the next round. It continues mercilessly, relentlessly, ruling your entire life. As powerful as drugs and alcoholism, it can take your family, friends, home and career and toss it all into a bin. If you finally realise the game is up, you might not then be in a good stable relationship or financial position to adopt, and adoption isn't what it should be. If adoption was not such a mind-blowing ridiculous ordeal I'm certain more people would choose adoption over IVF, or at least stop IVF and the heartbreak sooner. Adoption seemed to rule out good people, as some of my friends had learned, for trivial reasons; having a pet lizard, a hot tub, or too much decking and not enough grass – as if that couldn't be altered. Children from healthy pregnancies were, we were informed, hard to come by. It takes years for the paperwork to authorise a child for adoption which makes adopting a child under the age of three very rare. We had a responsibility to keep the biological parents updated annually and were informed that international adoptions were currently banned in the UK. I disliked the invasive ordeal all my friends and family would have to go through and I had seen better people than us messed around for years only to be disappointed. I even disliked being told I had to rip all my rose bushes up – I adored roses and couldn't understand such a stupid rule. My niece and nephew had special needs and I had watched the hard life my sister had led as a result. It was a very hard life to choose, far above the role of a parent, and although I would be the best mother I could if I had a child with special needs it was not something I would actively choose to do and I had great admiration for the selfless people who were better minded than I. Therefore, for a number of reasons, we ruled adoption out. IVF was easier, less humiliating and more private - strangely enough.

      We purchased a book on IVF and took it in turns to read a chapter to each other before bed until we had finished the book; *Couple's Guide to In Vitro Fertilization: Everything You Need to Know to Maximize Your Chances of Success* by Liza Charlesworth. It was brilliant for our relationship. It made us realise that we were blaming each other despite our pact; it made us understand each other's responses and made us feel connected to each other again. I was starting to get some scientific facts to help me understand this big complex procedure. I learned that by the time couples get to IVF they were exhausted, burnt-out, and negative: not a good way to start and I ensured we approached it as refreshed and as relaxed as possible. I also learned to understand James's denial attitude and why he refused to always do the things he was told to do – just like me with binge drinking and smoking actually – which was easy to stop once I had an IVF goal to follow. James opened up to me and said he had been blaming me too. That made me feel less shameful about being the same way – we were both doing the same thing. Upon this realisation our relationship improved. Decisions came easy for us – we would immediately think and choose the same – no added arguments or compromises for us when it came down to science. One of these decisions was whether or not to freeze embryos during the IVF cycle. We were happy with the possibility of twins. We could only have one or two embryos implanted so we went for two. Fresh embryos had a slightly higher rate of success than ones that had been defrosted so we decided not to pay the extra money to freeze them in this first instance. If it didn't work then we would do a fresh cycle of IVF next time.

***

The presentation was surprisingly busy with other couples who seemed as awkward as us as we gingerly munched biscuits with our tea and avoided eye contact. There was a silent understanding that no one would talk to each other and just pretend no one else in the room existed. The hospital had a good success rate of 49% considering they didn't screen their couples (some fertility clinics only take on couples most likely to conceive to keep their figures high). Two things remained with us to discuss on our car journey home. First, ICSI: it looked a rather harsh treatment of forcefully injecting the sperm into the eggs and I didn't like the idea of it. We were told that we might need it done and the knowledge gave me hope that I might be able to avoid it if we continued our extreme lifestyle that went beyond healthy. Second, the egg-donor scheme: if a woman doing IVF with no known problems was under thirty-five years old she could share her eggs. This helped another couple to potentially have a family and reduced our IVF costs. It made immediate sense to me. Most importantly, it made me feel so much more positive about the reason why I had to go through IVF – to give someone else a child. I could relate to that and it felt as if it were meant to be. We had already decided not to freeze any embryos the first time. This seemed like a sensible solution: save money, save wasting the eggs and give the gift of a child to someone else. It was something I instinctively wanted to do – it was a win-win all round.

The waiting list for donor eggs is currently three years at this hospital. My understanding was that these women may have gone through the menopause in their early or late thirties or numerous failed IVF rounds. They couldn't afford or didn't want to go abroad for eggs so were stuck in a country that didn't like to donate. Plus, they only got half a batch of eggs: either from the egg sharing scheme or if a woman gave all her eggs to the hospital they would be split between two women. They get one chance, or rather, half a chance. She was matched with me; same eyes, hair, build, even skill set. If it didn't work then she goes right back to the bottom of the three year waiting list – harsh! I realised that I could be that woman one day – who knew at this stage? I wanted to help. It wasn't as easy for eggs to be donated as it was for sperm and IVF was more expensive for those needing eggs. It hardly seemed fair. IVF was opening my mind to a different side of life. I started to realise how immature and lucky I was. I was beginning to understand what it was all about and felt my own personal anger at being deprived of a natural pregnancy shamefully trivial. I became aware of every miscarriage on the planet. I saw every pregnant woman on earth and some days it seemed as if everyone was pregnant – even double glancing at men with beer bellies! I kept switching the TV over just as a baby commercial came on or a woman in a film was giving birth. The world changed for me. I heard stories - not nice ones either. Everyone seemed to like making IVF horrible, either to scare you because they wanted someone else to suffer as much as they did, or because they want you to understand what hell they personally went through. Can IVF be discussed in any other way? It felt like I had to actively choose to walk along a bridge of mental cruelty after crossing a desert of physical infertility.

  The problem with donating eggs was that all the legal rights remained with the potential child (or more) and I personally thought the law had it all wrong. Any child created from my egg had the right to get my details when they reached the age of eighteen – if they wanted to – regardless of my situation or choice. It seemed unfair that someone who wasn't even alive got more rights than me. What about my choice and my family situation? We should be asked first. This was a major reason why so few people were currently donating in this country – the waiting list was huge – for both egg and sperm donors – the donor potentially facing future risks with changes in law. This was why the majority of people went abroad to purchase eggs or sperm, which were more readily available, with less risk, because donors were paid and laws were different. It was a lot to ask a woman to go through and they weren't compensated in any way in this country, which was hard when they need time off to attend appointments, recover, and risk their health and chances of having children themselves later on. Employers cannot carry the cost of such sick leave and should they have to? Small employers struggle already with things like maternity leave. However, technology constantly improves and less intrusive options were starting to become available but were currently limited to certain cases. Men still faced the same risk of being contacted later on but they had it far simpler; no time off, no health risks. The law constantly changed and didn't seem to reflect reality and I was worried that one day they might make donors financially responsible for any offspring. It can seem scary and I understood the reluctance. It was a tricky situation and I did't know the answer since paying a donor raises an entirely different set of moral problems.

One drawback I had was about the future of this offspring: what if the parents were in a tragic accident and the child or children ended up in care? I would like to be notified and be able to do something about that should it ever occur. This bothered me immensely. I would feel somewhat responsible for a child that could end up in foster care. How could I live with that? Would I ever have any reassurance that the life I helped create was going to be looked after properly and lovingly? I reluctantly pushed these negative thoughts aside, choosing instead to focus on the gift I would be giving and seeing the positive side. After all, it was still a life that otherwise wouldn't exist and I sincerely believed that a deprived child can and often do make more of their life than one born into riches. My own family life was traumatic, to say the least, and I escaped and survived it. In my experience, being biologically connected was overrated.

"What do you think?" I asked James as we drove home.

"It's completely your decision – they're your eggs," he replied.

"Yes, but it's our house some pent-up teenager can come banging down in eighteen years time."

"Your family is far worse, I'm more worried about them knocking on the door."

He had a good point. "My lot can find an argument in a mirror. But—"

"I'm not concerned in the least and imagine that anyone who got pregnant in this way would cherish the child and raise it accordingly."

"Should we do it?"

"Well, I want to just because of the money it saves but I didn't want to say anything in case you thought I was being cheap," he smiled.

"You are cheap and I knew that would appeal to you but you have to think beyond the money," I laughed.

We decided to take the counselling that explained more about it. We were told that we had the right mind-set and that we would qualify if we wanted to go ahead. I was encouraged by the comment that the counsellor made: "People who donate tend to have a higher success rate because of their age and the positive mind-set it gives you." I felt at peace with the idea that I had to face IVF so that I could help someone else and bring joy where it otherwise wouldn't be – the idea counteracted the cold science of what lay ahead. I was hooked.

The act of donating eggs didn't bother me at all. I had read enough history books to know that people had secretly slept with other people and had affairs to conceive when they couldn't with their married partner. IVF was a modern, honest and open way of confronting a natural dilemma. It sat comfortably with me. I just wanted and preferred a natural conception. I sometimes felt angry at God for giving us this unbearable yearning to have a child and yet prevent conception in such a cruel and cold manner. However, since I wasn't quite a Christian I couldn't hold on to that for long – how could I blame a God I didn't serve? Hypocritical, really. With the thought of donating and having an ulterior motive I felt the peace replace the anger within.

James had to provide another sperm sample and it was slightly better.

"If you provide a sample like this on the day then you won't need ICSI," the doctor said. "What we will do is place you on ICSI-backup so that we can make a final decision on the day as to whether or not we inject the sperm into the eggs."

"More green smoothies then," I smiled wickedly as he rolled his eyes in disgust.

We had to pay £1000 up front and would get it refunded if we didn't need to have ICSI. We were really pleased with this and

I felt justified in making James drink all those smoothies and do acupuncture – the two things that most bothered him. We will never know what really helped but it didn't matter – it looked good and we were set to go. I instantly regretted sharing the news with friends and family about egg donation and was shocked at some of their attitudes. I quickly realised what a highly sensitive and controversial subject it was. Naively, I thought this was something personal for us at this point in time, but it turned out that it was personal to everyone and stirred up many emotions in those around us. One would think it was their eggs I was giving away. I had the phone slammed down on me for giving away the nieces and nephews that *they* would never know. I had no other thought except that it was a kind and generous thing to do. I was still surprised that it was considered as "giving away babies." I was naturally very open, direct and honest. For the first time in my life, I thought very carefully about who I was with and what I said, which does not come naturally to me so I mostly avoided certain people. With each period, a woman creates and loses eggs, usually only maturing one egg from each monthly batch. Our body reabsorbs the rest, denying them life, being impossible to fertilise the thousands of eggs that each woman actually created in one lifetime. All IVF did was increase the amount of eggs reaching full maturity in one cycle and science helped me to keep things in perspective. It would be a completely different story, for me, if it were an embryo but I think even then I would rather help another person have a child than let an embryo fade into nothing. I decided negative viewpoints about donation didn't sit well with me or make sense and went back to my initial feelings and stuck with them. My instincts have never let me down. I tried not to think how gutted I would be if it didn't work – for them or for me.

Chapter 2 – The Dark Dingy Road Of Relentless Failing IVF

I was surprised by how positive and good I felt once IVF began: I had left infertility limbo and was actively doing something to change the situation. My drugs arrived and it began with the sort you sniff when you have a blocked nose. These had a horrible effect on me, unlike most of the other women I knew who suffered no side-effects. I was grateful to not be working: being in no fit state to do my job and far too emotional to hold a professional meeting. I didn't know why they affected me so much. I had menopausal symptoms: hot and cold sweats, bursting into tears for no reason, swinging from uncontrollable anger to deep melancholy – it was the worst thing I had ever experienced – I don't even suffer PMS. It had only just begun and I was petrified by the strength of the drugs and how rapidly they altered my nature. I couldn't hold a conversation and lost track mid-sentence, slurred or repeated sentences endlessly as if I were drunk, noticed more acutely by my friends. When I reached the stage of the injections I was beside myself and dreaded the moment all day long. I snuck off upstairs, not wanting to upset James with my fear. I placed a bag of frozen peas on the spot, as advised by the nurse, then proceeded to inject. I couldn't – my hand was shaking and I couldn't bear the thought of injecting myself even though the needles were tiny – like the ones diabetics use.

"Come on," I told myself, "kids with diabetes do this – you can do it!"

I couldn't.

My hand refused to respond, merely trembling over my stomach, as my dread of needles overcame me. James couldn't help; he was worse than me when it came to needles, and he'd probably end up hurting me more than I would myself. I called Jude, a friend I'd known since she had been my college lecturer. She was more like a mother to me but lived far away.

"You can do this," she told me in her no-nonsense manner. "You can do anything if you put your mind to it."

I told her I couldn't. I wanted to but fear had taken over and my hand refused to follow explicit instructions. I was not sure how long I was on the phone to Jude but she talked through that first injection – I will forever be grateful to her – as I have been for many reasons since I was seventeen. I cried, sweated, cringed and almost passed out and then, when it proved so painless and easy, I was thinking that perhaps I had done it wrong. It hadn't hurt at all, it was just about getting past that first one, and she got me there. Once I had done the injection I felt rather pathetic that I'd made a mountain out of a mole hill. I ran downstairs and told James how easy and painless it was, he was watching Battlestar Galactica and merely smiled, obviously dreading any further interruption to his program as he rudely turned up the volume. Such an emotional thing for me hadn't even reached him and I stood fidgeting next to him, wanting attention or conversation, and wondering what to do. He ignored me so I turned to my diary. After that, I breezed through the injections and had no side effects. James didn't like to see me go through this and felt guilty that he got off so lightly, especially because he considered the problem to be his. In truth, I grudgingly felt the same and only wanted him to acknowledge what I was going through and support me in what I had to do rather than leave me alone. I grew my own fruit and vegetables, ate good food, mostly raw, took supplements, exercised a lot, and rarely took medicine. My only downfall was my self-destructive behaviour inherited from a large family of smokers and drinkers, who lived on takeaways, sneered at the green stuff growing on a leg of lamb (rosemary) to the point of refusing to eat it, and saw fruit as something you only had at Christmas. I sometimes succumbed to these old habits when stressed. I wanted to be a better wife and have a good relationship again. However, there was a small part of me that was jealous of him having so little to do and perhaps it was his lack of support that made me feel this way. It felt like everything was on me and I didn't like it much. Once more I was aware of my whining ways and the unfairness that existed between men and women. I resented my body being subjected to such strong drugs and having to go through all this. "It's not fair" rolled around my vacuous head until it ached.

Despite these emotions, which I buried deep inside when meditation failed to purge the feeling, I tried to do the right thing. From that moment on, time seemed to speed by. I did the injections anywhere and in any room as if I was blowing my nose – it was that easy. I couldn't believe how worked up I had been and suffered minor side effects from these drugs. I had another scan and was really scared when some novice and inexperienced male nurse told me that I was overreacting to the drug and had OHSS (ovarian hyper-stimulation syndrome).This explained the bloating, shortness of breath, vomiting, calf, chest and lower abdomen pains. After a rather uncertain discussion in front of me, two nurses decided to just have me carry on and hope for the best. I left with the impression that they would have cancelled the procedure if I hadn't been sharing my eggs. There was no refund for all the cost, it was done on a "best effort" basis, and no one could guarantee anything. I'd often found it strange that with all our technology we knew very little when it came to fertility – it was pretty much all luck and guess work. Worse still, according to the list on the forms I had signed, I could be hospitalised with ruptured ovaries, lose a tube, end up having to have an emergency hysterectomy or worse. I did not trust their decision and was nervous leaving the hospital. However, I didn't want to make a fuss in case they treated me terribly from then on, and I already felt vulnerable. Another side of me told me to have faith in them, they were experienced, even if they didn't always seem it. It was a long couple of days but nothing bad happened.

The day came for the final big injection: Serono Ovitrelle taken precisely twenty six hours before follicle removal, if memory served me right. This injection would stimulate all my eggs to full maturity and it was essential that they were removed before this happened naturally otherwise my ovaries would rupture. I gasped in despair as I drew out the needle and saw the immense length of it in comparison to the others. I held an ice pack to my belly for twenty minutes before I had the courage to inject. The needle was long and there was a lot of liquid to push in. It seemed to take forever and made me queasy. My older sister had gone through IVF over a decade earlier and back then they did a massive injection in the thigh, leaving it black and blue for weeks: at least it had improved since. I had no idea, at this point, that I could have paid a little more for a smaller needle! I pushed the last bit of liquid in then pulled the bloody thing out as quickly as possible and lay in a cold clammy sweat. Finally, it was over. I had successfully completed all of the drugs on time and felt a large sense of achievement. I was as white as a sheet, trembling, and admittedly overly dramatic about it all. Now it was over, my work was done, and it no longer seemed such an ordeal. Once more I could not get James to comfort me. His way of dealing with IVF was to block it, along with me, from his everyday life as he drank wine and watched TV.

***

I wasn't worried about the egg retrieval since I wasn't expecting it to hurt immensely. I knew plenty of other women who hadn't felt a thing. Upon arriving at the hospital I could tell that the staff were edgy and nervous because of my overreaction to the drugs and I watched them grow increasingly worried about my health. I started to think they doubted their decision about making me continue with the drugs. They rushed me through and the first thing they did was scan me to find out how many follicles I had. I had a lot more water retention than normal and already looked eight months pregnant. I had over forty follicles but not all of them would contain the right size eggs. I lay on a bed with more people around me than I liked – about five – and had to open my legs. After a quick look down below and a few concerned glances they left the room to have a muffled conversation out of earshot. I was left lying there with my legs wide and high as I wiggled my fingers nervously. I knew they were worried about how bloated I was. I tried not to think about it – it was all out of my hands – I was getting better at giving up control. They left me alone long enough for me to have a quiet word with my follicles and the eggs they were holding. I placed my hand over my abdomen and spoke to them. I begged them not to let this be the last time we met, to come back to me and I would keep them warm and safe. It was the only time I showed any connection with them. The staff returned to the room and started to prepare me, obviously having decided they should go ahead, and began to prod and poke me down below - I felt violated – and was somewhat surprised at the inhumane way they were treating me. I felt like a slab of meat. I bit my lip and tried not to cry.

A very friendly anaesthesiologist injected me and talked to me as the procedure went ahead and she was great, although a little late, with distracting me from what was going on at the other end. I shall forever be grateful to her. They retrieved my eggs with something remarkably like a turkey-baster. I felt nothing at the time and chatted away with my usual nervous verbal diarrhoea as all the staff tolerated me with smiles and commented on how cute I was when drugged. I told them I was going to go home and do loads of ironing and they warned me to take it easy. I insisted I felt fine. In fact, I almost jumped off the table when it was over and they had to calm me down, laughing at me. I was so nervous and was putting on a brave face – they knew this. I joined James in the curtained off corner of a room while we awaited the results. I was starting to feel tired and before long I knew there was no way I'd be doing any ironing today or tomorrow. As the time passed, I felt more tired and low. We waited for the news as we watched the hands of the clock tick slowly around.

A couple in the next room to us, also curtained off so we could only hear, had a total of eight eggs to work with. It didn't sound like many to us and I began to think about my donated eggs, wondering what on earth I had done. I heard the nurse tell them that this was a good amount and they had two more than the last time. I felt sick, again wondering what I would do if I only had seven or eight and had to split them in half. I began regretting donating my eggs and felt sick with worry. On the other hand, if I didn't produce enough the poor woman I was donating to would be told that despite all the drugs and cost there wouldn't be any eggs for her – how heartbreaking! I had to produce six or more eggs to share – I could end up with only three. My mind was racing with conflicting emotions. I overheard another couple. I could tell from the conversation that she had problems producing eggs – even with the medication - she had got four this round and burst out crying.

"It's more than the last few times," the nurse soothed.

"It's still not enough," the woman said between sobs. "We won't have any to freeze again."

James and I looked at each other and he squeezed my hand. I swallowed hard as I listened to the gut-wrenching sobs. Just then, a very bubbly lady arrived to give us our news: there were seventeen viable eggs to be used, which meant nine for us and eight for our donor couple. The current average number of eggs each woman created was seven so this was excellent news. They would be graded and divided fairly between us – I wanted all the best ones and almost said so – I bit my tongue just in time. It took a while for the news to sink in and then for me to realise the sobbing had increased in the cubicle next to us - the woman had heard all our news just like we had heard hers. I was mortified – how awful for her to hear her four compared to my seventeen like that! She must feel terrible. It suddenly seemed inappropriate to have us all in the same room like this separated merely by curtains. I felt so sorry for that other woman. While I was having my eggs removed, James, and the donor's husband, provided a sample. James didn't feel awkward or weird; he just went into the little room and did his part. His sample was great; once it had been washed and freed from the surrounding fluid, which seemed to act like glue, so his sperm "livened up" and mobility improved, which meant that we didn't need ICSI: we would be getting a refund of £1000. At 13:00 his sperm and my eggs were put together in something like a Petri-dish, as were the donors. It was a big day for all four of us. It was all going well. Too well; a small nagging thought kept telling me and I tried to joke away my concerns about the staff getting the two men's samples mixed up.

***

I had to sleep sitting upright because my ovaries had filled with water and were so large and swollen I could barely move or breathe with the severe intensity of the pain – it was awful. I couldn't walk, sit or sleep. It was worse than anything I had so far experienced and all I kept thinking was this whole thing just kept getting worse. I kept telling myself that it was worth the pain to have so many eggs but my ovaries were too swollen and I was in unbearable agony. Self pity made it difficult to remain positive. We had to wait until 09:00 the next morning to find out if anything had happened. I couldn't shake the nagging feeling that this could all end up nowhere, we could end up right back at the beginning, waiting several weeks until I had a period or two before it was next safe to start the drugs again. It was a nerve-racking wait! I wondered if we should have just done the ICSI and forced fertilisation because we didn't yet know if my egg shells were too hard for his sperm to penetrate – being our first time we knew nothing. I regretted my desire to avoid ICSI for what suddenly seemed meagre reasons. This was all trial and error and because I was in too much pain to sleep the night passed slowly and painfully, allowing me far too much time to dwell upon my thoughts.

I was pacing the lounge by 8:30. By 9:00 I was near hysterical. James had gone to work and I paced, sipped water, and prayed not just for a phone call but for a positive one. By 9:10 I was close to tears but five minutes later the phone rang: five of our nine eggs had fertilised and we had to wait a further three days to see if they lasted. The next morning I rang up to check and was told one had died – we now had four embryos. We were extremely scared. I suddenly became very annoyed with myself for giving away those valuable eggs. I wanted my eggs back from that woman, who I had suddenly lost all sympathy for! I wanted more, I wanted them back, I could have snatched them from her. I could see my numbers going dramatically down: seventeen...nine...five...and now four. What was I thinking? I should have kept the lot! I didn't dare call again and just decided to see what the situation was on the Friday morning when we went in. With the immense pain and inability to sleep properly while upright, the days dragged slowly by.

***

Friday morning arrived and we nervously entered the hospital. I was terrified that all of our embryos had died. As we walked through the doors we could see an awful lot of gloomy faces in the waiting room – it had obviously been bad news for many couples. Some women were crying, some looked numb, some looked vacant. All the men seemed to have the same expressions – ghostly – regardless of their woman's response. We had got the last appointment of the morning and I hated the misery I saw all around me. In fact, the whole place had constantly seemed overly negative and miserable, especially the constant reminders not to expect too much or get too excited – I hated it. However, it was starting to dawn on me how many people they saw and devastated on a regular basis. Emma had even told me that many couples blame them when it doesn't work – as if they should have done something more – when they are trying their best. It was a difficult situation to be in because it was obviously one of the most intense and emotional things a couple could go through. I gulped, held James's hand and tried to look more relaxed than I felt. I followed Emma into the room and felt all my hopes plummet. I was told to wait on a bed and James sat next to me.

"You have four embryos, two of which are not good enough to be frozen so I suggest we forget about those and focus on the stronger two."

I gulped. Seventeen...nine...five...four...two – zero! It had happened so quickly and this was it.

"What grade are they?" I asked, pulling myself together, remembering all the information I had burdened my brain with over the weeks.

"We don't like to give out grades, we find it makes people more negative," Emma replied.

"Well, if you don't tell me I shall assume it is negative because the quality is really bad and you don't want to dishearten me. They tell you in America," I said.

She looked at me and blinked. I often get that reaction.

"I want to know," I insisted.

"Well, it means nothing, it's only the way we grade them."

"It means something when you grade them because you ensure only the strongest ones are put in and frozen – not wasting your time on the weaker ones because you know they won't survive the process. I have to know. I want to set my expectations accordingly," the way I looked at her was clear – I wouldn't back off.

"They change constantly and what they are today might not be what they are tomorrow. This is why if people have a lot of embryos to choose from we sometimes make them wait a day or two more so we can pick the strongest looking. However, in your case, you only have two. We would put the lower-graded two in if that was all we had to use and hope for the best—"

"You mean a miracle," I interrupted.

"If you like, yes. But you have two good ones so we aren't looking at a miracle at all."

"What grade."

She sighed. "You have a B and a C."

I gasped. "No A's?" It was like being back in school, always B's and C's, no matter how hard I worked. It was so frustrating.

"No, I'm sorry but like I said they change constantly and many babies have been born from B's and C's. It's when you reach the D and E area it gets harder to tell. But in saying that, many A's have been put in too and there has been no pregnancy. It really cannot be guessed – it's all luck. Just stay positive."

I felt sick. It had seemed like so many eggs only three days earlier. Just two mediocre embryos – that was it after all of this? I jealously wondered if the other couple had created an A.

I didn't like the way I was treated or having to fight for information as if I were a moron – I just wanted facts. I was merely a routine job and there was no warmth or empathy. It made me feel raw. Many of the staff lacked good social skills, to say the least, and I watched them offend numerous couples with their callous comments, while remaining oblivious to the hurt I could see on the people's faces. How could they not see it? For every ten sour-faced miserable nurses there was one really good one, whom I rarely got, so I was always pleased to see Emma. The news was being delivered in the kindest way possible and I liked Emma for that despite the reluctance to part with the facts. Other nurses were not as sociable. It was a shame because it was the most emotional thing I had ever had to go through and James and I were alone amongst a bunch of heartless professionals who didn't always seem to know what they were doing. I suppose they had to switch off their emotions to do this.

Our moment finally arrived. The embryologist stood out because she was so cheery and friendly, completely out of place compared to the other staff. But we were very grateful for her upbeat spirit and jokes – at least someone in this place was positive and unaffected by the atmosphere. I tried not to think about the two embryos we were ignoring. When a bitch had puppies she knowingly pushed a failing puppy aside, letting it die, while she focused on the ones she knew would live. I preferred the dog's more simplistic approach to life. I was merely focusing on the ones I knew would live and had no time for the ones that were barely sustainable. Harsh reality hit me: this was survival of the fittest. The coldness and distance of the staff started to penetrate through my skin and silent tears rolled down my cheeks. In reality I think it was simply the raw emotions making me cry and had little to do with the staff. What did I expect from them? A munchkin dance to cheer me up?

I asked if putting the embryos in would hurt – they said no – they were wrong. I was surprised by the pain and when I winced in agony the nurse coldly explained that I was still sore from the egg removal – it does hurt then! I hated that nurse who I'd not met before. James looked crushed. I felt it was all so unnatural and cold – what a way to conceive. He hated to see me in pain and could see how upset I was, silent tears pouring down my crumpled face, writhing and groaning in agony. Please God, don't make me go through all this again was all I could think. As we walked out I looked as glum and miserable as everyone else around me. There was something about this place where even good news was depressing and I was just another woman on the verge of tears, desperate to leave.

"Get me out of here now," I demanded through gritted teeth, fighting the pain.

James nodded and dragged me towards the stairs.

"No stairs!" I moaned.

He pulled me towards the lifts.

On the car journey home I tried hard to calm down and relax. I couldn't. I was hysterical – and all because I desperately needed a pee! There was nothing but a long country road with no bushes or cover and no open pubs or public toilets. I was literally crying in pain – there was no room for a full bladder with my swollen ovaries – and he was panicking because he couldn't find anywhere. It was ridiculous how stressful the car journey was – we both completely lost it – yelling insults at each other. He called me a moron for not using the toilets before we left the hospital and I called him an asshole for having a go at me instead of finding a toilet. I was in too much pain to think. Anyone watching us would find it hard to believe we had just experienced the wonder of two little lives being created. I cannot believe I made it to the house. I struggled up the stairs, holding myself as I sat on the loo, cringing and still crying with the sheer agony of passing water and terrified that I was peeing the embryos out – even though I'd been told it wasn't possible. It was horrendous. Tears rolled down my cheeks as I gripped the bath, spasms of pain intermittently stopping the flow of pee.

The pain was so bad all I could do was stay in bed sobbing. This part was unexpected, it was not supposed to hurt and I didn't know anyone else who had found it painful. I later learned that it was because I'd been over stimulated. I didn't want to be different in this particular area. The next morning I awoke refreshed and more myself. Two women arrived, as scheduled, to perform reiki and acupuncture on me. It was lovely. Their kindness an support was a breath of fresh air and they knew just what to say. I immediately started meditating, an IVF meditation I had purchased, and visualising happy growth; trying to undo any damage I had done the day before. I checked my pants constantly for signs of blood. James slipped into depression because he said there was absolutely nothing he could do now – it didn't matter what he did or how healthy he was – his part was over. I reminded him that this was not strictly the case as he could focus on looking after me and make sure I kept rational – my hormones didn't know what had hit them! We were both immensely relieved, at the end of the IVF cycle, compared to how we were at the beginning. I was telling myself to be calm and was absolutely petrified of messing this up at such a late stage. What if they didn't stick? What if they fell out? What if I was not pregnant in two weeks time? I had cried upon starting many periods in the past but this time I knew that I had two fertilised embryos in me. I knew I was pregnant. All I could do was pray and hope. I was unable to stop looking at baby stuff to buy and a nagging voice told me not to get my hopes up.

Walking Fudge prevented me from going stir-crazy. I took her to the beach, longing to see the ocean, desperately trying to manage my anger and fury. The outrage of having a natural conception stolen from me still bothered me immensely along with suffering financial cuts others don't have to make. Fudge gave me unconditional joy, love, and company that got me through. On really bad days I would let her come and lie on my bed with me. If I was sad she would comfort me. I really felt that she understood and she was constantly sniffing my stomach and I knew she could detect the embryos. I kept my days simple but found relaxing hard to do. At first I redecorated the whole house, re-stained any outside wooden furniture I could find, even my neighbours, in order to justify not working. It was a culture shock for me. I had worked since I was eight, washing up in my parents hotel. It took months to learn to relax. I played with the chickens in the garden, cuddled the cats and bought new fish – as many as my little BiUBE tank could handle. I kept very busy. The second week was easier: halfway there and no blood. I felt more positive. I felt pregnant and Fudge was still detecting the embryos. James started cycling and I pretended not to care – ignoring the nagging thought in the back of my mind about what if this didn't work and he was damaging his sperm bank once more. It infuriated me but I said nothing. I wanted to avoid confrontation.

I was on the sofa lying down, feet in air, when the phone rang. It was a friend I hadn't spoken to for a while. She knew I was going to do IVF but was not in my close circle of friends so had no idea when or how it was going. She didn't know that the embryos had been placed in only three days earlier. I cried as I listened in silence to the story of the abortion my friend had just experienced and how similar it was, the procedure, to my IVF in some ways. It was awkward and our situations were worlds apart. This was the first friend I lost – we never fell out – we just never bothered talking to each other again.

***

The two week wait after the embryo transfer dragged; we were like zombies, didn't know what to do with ourselves apart from feel awful. A day would pass and we'd realise that we hadn't got anywhere or done anything. During the second week eczema broke out on my calves and I felt queasy and light headed – then I was certain I was pregnant. Wednesday, the day before our pregnancy test, was strained to say the least. I was so moody and wound up I even burnt two fingers while boiling pasta. I cried a lot. James came home from work and looked as if he was going to puke – he almost did while brushing his teeth that night. Sleep was impossible.

I gave up trying to sleep and declared, "I'm going to do it."

"It's barely five, it's too early," he replies sluggishly.

"I can't wait any longer. Today is the day – they never said at what time."

What could he say? I got out of bed, walked into the bathroom, piddled on the stick and returned with it held like the Olympic torch. I crawled into bed, placed the stick on the bedside table, so very carefully and upright, and we cuddled as the time passed. James stared blankly at the ceiling as I watched the blink...blink...blink... of the digital clock on the bedside table. Finally, I rolled over to look at the results. James did not turn with me. He saw the huge smile on my face and it devastated him - he thought I was in for the biggest disappointment of my life and he covered his eyes with one arm and sunk back into his pillow. I beamed with excitement – I knew I was pregnant. I had to be. Every instinct in me was adamant and all doubts had gone. James saw this on my face and dreaded my reaction more than the actual results. I stared at the stick. I blinked. My eyes blurred as tears welled up. He wouldn't look at me and remained lying on his back, arm over his eyes, waiting for the hysterical sobs. It took a while for me to compose myself enough to speak. He must have felt terrible and had no idea that I was waving the stick at him while I tried to form words.

"Pos-positive," I finally managed to splutter before bursting into tears of joy.

His arm jolted away from his eyes and he sat bolt upright.

"Are you fucking kidding?" he gasped.

"I'm fucking pregnant!" I sobbed and we clung to each other, shaking and crying, until dawn finally broke.

It was the beginning of December. I had my greatest wish – I was pregnant – I was getting a baby – possibly two! I was pregnant for the Christmas holidays.

Chapter 3 – Darren and Julie

Darren was twenty five, Julie aged sixteen when they began playing in the same band: Julie played the keyboard and Darren the guitar. They had no intention of dating and played together for a couple of years, even sharing a flat together with Darren's current girlfriend. Julie continued to live with Darren's ex-girlfriend after their separation. They continued to commute to rehearsals together. It was a few months later when they started dating. They were party animals and often out until the early hours of the morning. On one such morning, at six o'clock, they were having a mild argument when Darren suggested they get married. They cannot remember how it happened or what they were arguing about. Darren had seen ample bed-hopping and relationship-hopping to know it wasn't his thing.

"I hold the same Victorian values as my father and knew this felt right. I'm the sort of person who rides the storm and doesn't run away – problems toughen you up. My parents went through a lot of rocky times but forty years later they're still going strong," Darren explains.

The date wasn't important and after a few joking comments that they might select February 29th so that they only had an anniversary every four years they decided to run with it. They married on a Tuesday in a registry office.

"It was the statement we wanted; not the certificate, expense or show of a big wedding and we wanted to avoid the falseness of a church since we weren't religious," Darren said.

Since they played in pubs and clubs they chose to have their reception in a pub with a finger buffet and hot pasties direct from Cornwall, where his family originated from.

"We refused to have any cheesy wedding music, it was all scar and two-tone music and we even surprised everyone with our first dance – one step beyond by madness. Everyone got up to dance, not just us, and it was great," Darren smiles.

"It was a nice relaxed event and people dropped by to share a drink with us," Julie adds.

"It was a very memorable evening and everyone said how different and nice it was – none of the boring speeches and formality of a normal wedding."

Darren is an identical twin and during the wedding his mother accidentally threw confetti over Julie and Darren's identical twin, which they still laugh about.

"She was so caught up in the moment," Darren laughs.

"It was a bit odd but so funny," said Julie.

The wedding cake collapsed as they cut into it and they merely laughed – nothing stressed or fazed them on their wedding day. It was a light-hearted fun day – just what they had wanted. They went to Rome for a holiday and were in no rush to have children. It was during another holiday in Greece when things changed. Darren experienced sudden panic attacks: heart racing, he would stop abruptly in the middle of the street, eyes swimming and wonder where he was. It was scary and at one point he thought he was having a heart attack and was going to die. Darren had never before experienced anything like this and it had come out of nowhere. One attack lasted nine hours and he had several during the holiday. They had been married for two years and this is what got them thinking about the long term and wanting children. Upon their return to England, Darren visited a psychologist who said this was deferred reaction to something in his past and he was able to overcome it. For the next eighteen months they tried to get pregnant while a number of problems entered their lives. Darren's health was one problem he was overcoming and one evening they and two other people were victims of an unprovoked attack – a group of teenagers on drugs brutally assaulted them. It shocked them that something like this could happen and was incredibly difficult to overcome. Darren started drinking heavily and was often drunk. Julie then began to have health issues and started fainting. She was taken away in an ambulance and told it was a urinary infection. She stopped drinking; suspecting alcohol was making her feel sick, but nothing improved. She was starting to get angry about not falling pregnant and her health was deteriorating. After another ambulance journey they discovered that she had endometriosis, a large cyst, and was given drugs to take that would stop her periods, along with her ability to get pregnant, for a year.

"I didn't want us to be one of those childless couples spending their whole lives trying desperately for a child, it's so sad, and wanted to go away for a year and forget about it all," Julie said. "We decided to go to Spain for the year while I was taking the drugs."

Darren gave up a good promotion, realising how much Julie needed to get away, and putting their mental wellbeing first. Upon their return to England, Julie stopped the drugs and soon blacked out again. She was referred for IVF because of the endometriosis. Julie wasn't sure what to expect and assumed that she would be treated on the NHS. After the initial consultancy she was shocked when they shoved a pricelist under her nose.

"They coldly told me that because I was only twenty nine I couldn't be treated on the NHS, despite my endometriosis preventing a natural conception, and stuck what seemed like a Chinese menu under my nose," Julie says as she rolls her eyes in disbelief. "I hadn't even considered that I would be buying my baby and what the cost would be. All I could see was large figures and I went as white as a sheet – I was speechless."

Since the violent attack, they decided to move area and live in the country. They could use some money from the house sale for IVF and spend less on their next purchase. It was not ideal but at least it was possible. Darren felt immediately relaxed in the country and the move completely changed their attitudes and life – especially his.

"I find it difficult that there is a post code lottery with this sort of thing," he tells me. "If we had lived in a different area we could have had IVF on the NHS – Julie had an illness preventing pregnancy. I don't like the fact that it's done on what County you live in – we all live in the same country and all cover each other's costs. Our taxes cover everyone else's NHS treatment so why could some areas accommodate people like my wife and not the one we lived in? I found that hard to understand."

"Since we had no choice and were going to have to pay for it privately we decided to shop around," Julie said.

"I didn't like the way we were treated. It was like walking into a shop; no sympathy, no support and nothing personal about it – just how much to buy your baby," Darren added.

They did some research and were curious that many of the clinics had a 25% success rate but one had a startling 55% success rate. It was more money, intense monitoring but almost guaranteed success and since they only had one shot at IVF, due to financial reasons, it was worth going for. Julie would have a long commute into London each day for monitoring and had to tell her boss. Despite working flexi-hours and being open about it, her boss was rude and non-supportive.

"He had his second kid on the way and had no sympathy for me. He even wrote a really long nasty email saying I was taking the piss. I was doing all my hours, just around the appointments. It wasn't very nice," Julie sighs.

To make matters more complicated, just as they started with the drugs, the clinic was all over the news and Panorama. Many friends and family told Julie and Darren to avoid the clinic. Police barged into the clinic to search for documents.

"All I could think about was how the poor people mid-IVF must have felt, especially those in the clinic at the time of the search. It was so insensitive. They could have done it better and not put all those people through that," Darren said.

"The clinic was really busy, almost like a conveyor belt, and the consultant oversaw every single case – he was very popular and successful," said Julie.

"We watched the Panorama documentary, wondering what on earth the guy had been up to and not knowing what to expect, but it was obvious to me what was going on. I am a scientist and could see he was pushing scientific boundaries and getting excellent results. It was nothing bad and the people against him on

Panorama allegedly had a vested interest in seeing him go down and lose clients: apparently, they had IVF clinics with much lower success rates."

"They accused him of not having a license, which was exaggerated because it was only for about a month and what could he do while there was an unexpected delay in the renewal – cancel all those people in the middle of IVF? He was only without a license for a month, it wasn't as bad as they made out."

"It was edited in a shocking way," Darren nods.

"Loads of people were really angry, he was a good man, and they protested outside his clinic on his behalf. We didn't feel bad about staying with him at all. In fact, it made us more positive and determined to have our IVF with such an innovative man."

"They tried to make him out as some sort of a Maverick but he just excelled in what he did and the competition didn't like it. That's all I could see," said Darren. "It was difficult because people kept on at us to not go with them but they are not scientists, like me, and didn't understand. We knew him, felt comfortable, and were more than happy."

They were given little yellow back packs full of drugs to carry with them, identifying his clients, they laugh, and Julie proudly took hers everywhere. Darren couldn't believe how Julie travelled to London daily, up long before him and returning late each night after work, receiving daily monitoring and information on what dosage of drugs to take each day.

"I was gobsmacked by her perseverance and overwhelmed by her endurance," he tells me proudly.

She commuted far to London, daily, for six weeks, including weekends and as a result of the monitoring she had no adverse reactions to the drugs at all and carried on as normal. Julie was terrified of needles and couldn't bring herself to do the injections. Darren did them for her, when she was at home, and a supportive and enthusiastic colleague did them at work. Julie breezed through IVF, determined to reach her goal, and didn't complain at all. She secretly dreaded every day because of that injection she would have to face on the evening but was perfectly relaxed once it was done – until the next day. Darren didn't realise this as she hid it well at the time.

"I was really scared of OHSS," Darren admits.

"Me too," Julie agrees.

"It was something I was scared would happen to her but she wasn't over stimulated at all and wasn't in any pain even when they harvested the eggs."

"I was told to drink four litres of water and loads of milk each day, which I found hard to do, it was a lot of fluid. That was the only pressure I remember."

They had nine eggs: seven fertilised, two were put in and only one was strong enough to be frozen.

"I did my part after staring out of the window for ten minutes. It was all just part of the process, like cutting your toe nails but different because cutting your toe nails wasn't as important. After all we had been through – a lot depended on this," Darren explains. "I didn't like being put on the spot and given only an hour to decide whether we paid the huge price to have one egg frozen. I didn't expect that. It was difficult to make such a decision at such short notice and we had no idea whether the two placed in would work. We felt forced to say yes."

Their anniversary, a leap year, was the day of fertilisation and they stayed overnight in a hotel. They had not been able to look at the forms and complete all the difficult questions, such as what would happen to the embryos if one or both of them died. They did it almost carelessly and in a rush because it was too hard to face. Julie feels bad about this because it was important questions and she felt that they should be taken more seriously. It was too much for them at the time. The two week wait was very hard after so many appointments and then nothing – just far too much time to keep her feet up and wait. Julie would struggle with basic concepts such as emptying the dishwasher and whether it would put the pregnancy in jeopardy – she had been told to keep her feet up – but for how long? Unable to wait the entire two weeks, Julie did an early test and it was negative. She prepared herself for the worst. When the two weeks were over she travelled first thing into London for the pregnancy test and had her blood taken, expecting to return home and wait for the results. Instead, they told her to wait because if she was pregnant then they would give her further drugs to take during the pregnancy. This was unexpected and Julie didn't know what to do with herself; she went shopping and purchased things she couldn't afford in an attempt to occupy her mind. Going almost insane, she called Darren and learned that his twin brother was in London and could meet her for coffee. By midday, sipping coffee with her brother-in-law, she rang the clinic and learned that she was, indeed, pregnant. Julie concealed her emotions because she didn't want Darren's brother, sitting opposite, finding out first. She called Darren and shared the good news. The clinic gave her different injections and told her to inject twice a day for the first twenty weeks of her pregnancy: once in her bottom and once in her stomach. This was an unexpected cost and they hadn't budgeted for it. Each injection was approximately £100.

"It was very difficult for me to inject her bump as it grew tighter and I was terrified of hurting the baby," Darren said. "Each injection created scar tissue and bumps so I had to keep finding a new place to do it. It was hard and scary. We stopped, at twelve weeks, when the bump got too big and because we couldn't afford it."

"It optimised the chances of a healthy pregnancy, because we had never been pregnant before and didn't know how likely we would be to miscarry, but twenty weeks was a long time," Julie adds.

Their scans were amazing and Julie remembers seeing the facial features of her baby. They decided against knowing the sex and waited until the birth. Her pregnancy was enjoyable. When she was two weeks overdue something felt odd and she asked Darren to take her into hospital. Initially, she thought she was imagining being in labour because she wanted to avoid being induced and had no pain and only an unusual odd feeling.

"Giving birth was something I wanted to do naturally since the baby wasn't conceived that way," Julie explains. "I didn't want to be induced."

"She was so calm I didn't think she was in labour at all," Darren said.

Upon arriving at the hospital, Julie learned that she was already seven centimetres dilated and five hours later Tara arrived. She had a glass of wine with paracetamol at the beginning of labour which helped relax her.

"I was peeved," Darren admits, "because it happened so fast I didn't even have time to have a blast on the gas and air!"

The midwives were very clean and efficient and they received great attention. Darren did not enjoy the birth because he was run down with a cold and sneezing and coughing everywhere. He was paranoid about passing on his germs.

"I really _really_ enjoyed the birth," Julie smiles. "Every bit of it even though I got carted off in an ambulance at the end because I had a bad tear high up."

"You were really high so that didn't bother you – you weren't in pain – you were smiling away! I had Tara in the van, following you in the ambulance, and kept thinking *"Bloody hell!"* I was suddenly having to protect and look after her. It was the best moment of my life."

They found it very tough at first and Darren was ill for the first few weeks, his panic attacks returned for a second time with a vengeance and it was hard to overcome. He was told it was as a result of all the stress and now that their goal had been achieved it was all coming to the surface. He bounced back quick enough and soon relished fatherhood. It had all been overwhelming – the whole long process – not just IVF but the illness and attack during their infertility time. He was also juggling a new job. It was an emotional time. Julie also struggled from the start, especially with breastfeeding.

"During pregnancy I almost imagined holding my baby to my breast while butterflies fluttered above us but it was so hard to establish. I was walking around the hospital topless and crying my eyes out, unable to feed my baby. It wasn't how I imagined it to be."

The pressure of midwives saying one thing and conflicting information at every turn was difficult to understand. Tara had night terrors and sleep was hard to find. It was really tough and Julie often wondered what on earth she had done. She wasn't great at routine and found it all much harder than expected.

"IVF was easy compared to afterwards," Darren said.

Julie nods. "I felt guilty for finding motherhood so tough. I had a lot of morbid thoughts at first, it was quite a dark patch, and it made me feel so bad because I was supposed to feel happy."

"But it's great now," Darren interrupts. "I think about Tara and Julie every day and it's fantastic."

"Yes, it was just the beginning. Then we loved everything about it."

One year later the clinic called to ask if they wanted to pay the renewal on refreezing the embryo. Darren is not just a scientist but a realist and he knew the chances of this one embryo working was slim. Two fresh ones, of a higher quality, had been implanted and only one had taken so this embryo, lower in quality and weakened due to the freezing, was unlikely to produce life no matter how much money they threw at it. They made the very difficult decision to let it go.

"So many people can argue about the humanity of the decision but it is yours to make," he said. "It's a personal decision. The embryo was only a grade five out of ten - it wasn't a life – it was a double cell."

"I was also worried about placing far too much hope on this one little embryo then being too upset if it didn't work. We had Tara and were happy with that. We had created life and had a family," Julie added.

"I don't think of Tara as an IVF baby at all unless someone reminds us how long we were married for before we had her," Darren explains. "That's the only time I think about it."

"I think about IVF more and still see her as an IVF baby."

"Julie went through IVF physically but we both went through it emotionally and financially – the men have to deal with it too," Darren sighs. "It's the fact that we could have had it on the NHS if we had lived somewhere else that peeves me. It makes people suffer and go through too much. I was never resentful of anyone else's pregnancy, even when my twin brother married after us and they fell pregnant on the honeymoon; I held no resentment at all. It's just the way it is. What I didn't like was how other people felt awkward around us and concealed things. It was obvious and I didn't like that at all."

"I think IVF cost us too much money and took away any backup or option for me to stay at home with Tara. I have to work full time and went back early. We were broke. Sometimes I resent what it cost."

Darren often drops Tara off at preschool and is enjoying looking after his ladies. He looks very happy. Julie is now thirty four: a very young age in the world of IVF.

Chapter 4 - Divine Pregnancy: Here they come

I went to my GP to share the good news and she did another pregnancy test for me there and then. I sighed with relief. Upon seeing my face my lovely doctor did two more pregnancy tests.

"You can never see the results or hear it too often," she smiled, genuinely enjoying my expression.

It was confirmed. I was walking on air. I was pregnant. The emotions that raged within me, releasing all that had happened, embracing what was happening, were undeniably chaotic and I loved it. It had been such a heavy program of drugs, timings, visits and now I just had to live normally and wait. I didn't know how to do that and didn't know how to fill the days for a while. I was often tired and hungry. I had really bad sinus congestion which turned into a lot of sneezing, nose blowing, coughing – it almost seemed like a winter bug. My body was exhausted and emotionally I was drained. I slept through Christmas – literally. I was awake for a mere three hours on Christmas Eve. It just all hit me. Eventually, I began to feel elated, healthy and pregnant. I needed to eat little and often to keep the queasiness at bay and when I wasn't hungry or couldn't stomach food I forced raw fruit and vegetables down. Luckily, there was no vomiting. My GP had booked us a midwife appointment for later in January.

I was adamant it was twins; I felt it in my heart. Their star signs should be Leo - I had already nicknamed them my little lion's. We had beaten the odds and gotten pregnant in half a round of IVF. This had been the best Christmas of my life; we had already planned to spend it alone as a couple knowing it was going to be a very good or a very bad time and hoping it might be our last one together. What a beautiful end to the year. The relief was marvellous.

The Labrador Retriever was often trained to sniff out tumours, cancer, diabetes and epilepsy (the chemical changes they induce) and I could see why – Fudge had known from the start that they were there and I shared my pregnancy with her. James was surprisingly distant and I really missed his company. I put it down to his way of dealing with the emotional shock of it all but I felt so very alone – swinging from feelings of elation and terror. No one called me and I felt as if I had no one to talk to and no friends for a while. I didn't realise everyone was just giving me some space to settle down. It was hard to keep my chin up and get through each day. I desperately wanted the company of my friends but they were busy with their careers or going out. I had all this excitement and joy and no one to share it with. Having worked abroad and in London, I knew nobody local. I couldn't understand why James was so withdrawn.

***

It was not a great start to the morning. Chi Chi, my Siamese cat, dragged me from my dreams by attempting to puke on my head. I awoke to push her off just in time. However, it was not soon enough to prevent spillage on my pillow. Not one for missing the opportunity for food, Fudge made a fast move for the puke and started to wolf it down. At this point I was retching. The dog wasn't normally on our bed but we had just decorated the dining room and I didn't want her sleeping downstairs with the fumes. James couldn't possibly stay asleep with all this commotion so woke up and helped me. He cleaned up the puke while I held Fudge off and we stripped the bed. Chi Chi was nowhere to be seen and I was not worried about her – she often gulped her food down too quickly then puked – just not normally on me. She had been acting strangely since I became pregnant and I was amazed at how intuitive the animals were. James went back to sleep but both the smell and the trauma lingered for me – I was terrified that such stress would cause a miscarriage so got up to do some yoga and meditation. I fed Chi Chi and Gemma (my obese Tabby), Fudge and let her outside for her business while I let the chickens out then made a cup of tea. At last, a bit of peace and quiet and it was barely 05:30. I watched the news and sipped my tea. We were, apparently, slumping into an economic depression; many jobs had been lost right on Christmas, poor Honda had to pull out of racing because they couldn't afford the 200 million a year or some ludicrous amount of money. It was unrealistic to me, spending such money on vehicles when it could be spent on people and animals, and I failed to understand the attraction compared to the cost. The news was overwhelming with negativity and depression - I turned it off. What could I do now? I was not used to so much time on my hands.

I got up to refill my tea and Fudge charged energetically upstairs and jumped on the bed. I heard James scream like a girl. She must have landed on his head with those sharp clumsy feet. I should let him sleep. I was far from considerate at the moment: my brain was like mashed potato. James always seemed to come unstuck with the pets: they were great with me but they somehow seemed to aggravate him. Chi Chi delivered little sandpaper licks to his eyeballs when he was asleep. I found it hilarious watching him flinch until he woke up and realised what is going on. Many times I had buried my face in the pillow, hiding the giggles and pretending I was still asleep. Sometimes the cat would even lick his bald head until it went red raw. He would get so angry and I would cry silently with laughter – often convinced the animals tormented him for my personal entertainment. This was why I adored animals and their funny little ways. I especially loved it when she sat on his chest and glared down at him.

"That cat is possessed!" he would screech almost hysterically when he awoke and saw her. "She's freaking me out and putting some sort of curse on me."

It was also the times she would stare at the wall and her eyes would dart everywhere watching something that wasn't there, as cats do, and as Siamese do most eerily.

"What the hell is she doing?" he would ask.

"She's watching dead people," I'd respond calmly.

"Oh, shut up!"

"Seriously, they can see the other side. You don't see anything do you? Well, she does – there's obviously someone there – look at the way her eyes are moving – she's watching someone."

It scared him to death and all the colour would drain from his face. He loathed horrors; I sometimes dared him to watch one with me, a mild one by my reckoning, and he would draw blood on my hand or hide behind me. I had a rather expensive collection of rare porcelain dolls I'd collected since I was thirteen and they are all boxed up in the loft because I wasn't allowed to have them in the house – they scared him. The animals ruled him but he refused to do anything I suggested to prevent it from happening. I don't know why, it wasn't hard to set a hierarchy and let them know who was boss: I'd never found it a problem, and he had pets when he was a child. However, he was in boarding school from the age of five so probably had little to do with them. He wasn't the sort to get down and play with a dog. He hated me suggesting anything to him and ignored my advice so the dog takes him for a walk and the cats tormented him. This, I decide, leaves me with no other choice but to enjoy the funny side of it, even if he can't, although he has loved the animals for years. James can be funny, hilariously so, when he likes, but not with the everyday things and with the last few years our humour had all but vanished.

***

I was in my 6th week. My happiness increased with each passing day. We waited in the hospital for our names to be called for our first scan, holding hands so tightly it hurt. We were nervous and fidgeting, scared they would tell us that the pregnancy wasn't viable. Since we had paid privately, we were seen on time. My legs trembled and I immediately began senseless ramblings as I talked my way into the room. All our hopes and dreams could be shattered at any moment. Emma managed to make me feel comfortable. She had been up all night with her young sick toddler and was exhausted. It didn't faze me – I longed to be kept up all night for such a reason. Strange how I remembered what she said but not a word of what I uttered during my bout of verbal diarrhoea. I lay down and tried to hide how much I was shaking, especially my arms and legs, as she rubbed the gel over my belly. Finally, a scan that wasn't internal. James and I had not let go of each other's hands – mine had gone numb - I guessed his was too. I heard his breath shakily escape from his lips, his only sign of nerves, as I shook and remained vividly aware that my mouth didn't stop moving with idiotic words. Emma smiled at me; she thought it cute, she said, but I felt like an idiot and couldn't be quiet. She placed the scanner on my belly and I saw images begin to flash upon the screen. I finally fell silent. I didn't dare breathe. I swallowed hard and watched her frown with intensity. She turned to me, still frowning. She didn't look as if she was about to deliver good news.

"Just tell me," I said tearfully, unable to make sense of anything on the screen through my blurred eyes.

"It's OK," she said, taking my free hand and finally replacing the frown with a smile. "You are pregnant. I can see them both clearly - look."

The word "both" gave me goose bumps. I vaguely remember her going on to mention something about how people don't really understand that the number of embryos means the number of children you get because so many people have two or three implanted and only have one baby. All I saw was her smile and I caught up with the conversation when she began pointing to the screen and showing me the tiny butter-bean images and explaining how two were babies and two were placentas and that they were the healthiest type of twins you could ask for. I let out a long shaky breath and tried to maintain some composure. James breathed a sigh of relief, bowing his head and squeezing my hand until I thought he would crush it.

"I take it you are both happy with the idea of twins?"

We nodded.

"Many pregnancies begin with twins and people never realise because they lose the second baby within twelve weeks, before the first scan is done. The likelihood of you losing both is slim so for your own sake do not get too focused on having more than one."

I completely ignored her and immediately began thinking of names for the twins – names I would never be able to use if I lost one – but I wouldn't let myself think that way. Fudge continually sniffed my stomach and located two separate entities each time. As long as she did that I knew both babies were there.

***

We had another scan at eight and twelve weeks. We could see their little sacs, their head and limbs and their heartbeats pounding – it was amazing. James had to go back to work and called me constantly because he couldn't concentrate – it was lovely to see him happy at last. I don't think we had ever felt such happiness. One moment I was furious at having to go through IVF and envisioned years of a battle, the next minute we were the easiest IVF case I had heard of. We had been unusually lucky: it made me scared that it was too good to be true. I browsed on line all day for twin things I might like, signed up to a couple of things, well, a lot of things actually, and brought some baby and pregnancy books. James told his parents and brother, I told friends and siblings. Everyone was over the moon at us having twins because there were none in our immediate network. It was exciting but it was going to be hard on my body and the first year after birth was not something I was really looking forward to – I would just be a milk pump and a nappy changing machine – I won't even have time for a bath, I'll barely be able to fit in my own toilet breaks. This was what I was being told at the twins club.

We keep looking at the photo from the scan and could not believe our luck or get our heads around it all. FABULOUS. I didn't like people who constantly went on about the risks. I was aware that I might lose one, yes I could miscarry, yes I might not make it to the end of the pregnancy or through child birth – I was not an idiot – but why constantly bring it up? It was not going to make me any less miserable if it happens but some people seem to think it will be easier to bear if they talk about it all the time. There was little balance; all negative predictions and not enough positive. I wanted to relish the joy I felt radiating through my body – over the years I had forgotten what joy felt like. People constantly voicing the risks were ruining my moment and dampening my spirits so I learned to avoid the people with negative attitudes or, as they claimed, realistic ones. I adored being pregnant. I occupied myself with exercise, training Fudge, creating a family tree photo album for the twins (which was harder than I imagined because no one remembered anything in their sixties and seventies!) and my 'Waiting for babies' memory album. On the first page I choked up as I wrote the following:

My greatest wish, hope, dream has at last come true... I am to be a mother of two wonderful little gifts xxx

I had problems with my pelvis right from the start, not just being tilted but the shooting pain. My history of sciatica and neuritis weigh heavily upon my mind but I walked the dog for two hours every day and maintained my daily yoga to keep strong. All I could hope was that my body wouldn't fail me at this crucial stage. I felt confident that I would cope. Only my back problems worried me. I had always suffered with bouts of depression after a serious episode of sciatica: not clinical depression but the sort brought on by frustration, constant pain and sleep deprivation and had alternative medicine to eliminate it back in my twenties. It had begun aged nineteen. There had been one time, aged twenty six, before I met my husband, when I was particularly scared by it all. Getting ready for work one morning, I bent down to pick my laptop case up and couldn't get back up. It took me an hour to get through the pain of moving slowly and carefully to reach the phone to call work and tell them that I couldn't come in. I then lay on my back and proceeded to call every supermarket in the area to see if someone could drop me off some cat food and basic supplies – not until tomorrow – you have to order on line 24 hours in advance. I explained that I could not sit at a computer or wait twenty four hours to feed my cats and would pay any of their staff £50 if they would drop me a bag of shopping off after their shift – would they please ask? No, on grounds of protecting their staff from strange people, and my argument about temporary disability went unheard. I received a firm "no" from everyone as if I was some psychopath. Was there no kindness in the world?

I kicked myself for being so disorganised and leaving everything to the last minute, which was something I've never allowed to happen since. It was typical that I was supposed to pick up cat food on my way home from work that day. I painfully searched for some tinned fish and couldn't believe I didn't have any. I lived alone, rarely cooked, ate out or skipped meals and my cupboards were bare. It suddenly became blatantly obvious to me that I had no one I could call upon. All my family and friends lived at least ninety minutes away, they all worked, and they were all too busy. I had only just moved here for my job and had not established any friends or met any civilised neighbours. I was terrified.

After a few hours, covered in deep heat and reduced to overdosing on pain killers, I walked out of the house to the local pet shop. It was a fifteen minute walk each way, I was incapable of driving, and each step pinched my sciatic nerve sending excruciating pain down my leg. Tears of pain ran down my cheeks and I held myself as steady as I could. It took forever and everyone stared at me. I looked like a lunatic on day release with the way I walked and cried to and from the pet shop with increasing humiliation. I was house-bound for five days, not moving off the floor in the lounge except to go to the toilet, feed the cats and myself: which happened rarely to limit the amount of pain I had to go through. I felt so alone and scared in the world. A year of hell and ineffective treatment followed but it was bearable because that was also the year that I met my husband. I learned to take the pain, resolved most of the issues so that I could lead a relatively normal life and gradually improved. I began to gain weight because I could no longer exercise and the new man in my life was an excellent cook who loved feeding me up and offering me far more wine than I should like. We were happy. My orthopaedic surgeon wasn't very good, gave me an epidural so that a group of surgeons could man-handle me back into place, which disabled me for over a month and only made matters worse. The physiotherapist saw me twice a week, more as a regular earner than someone to help, and nothing came of a year of these visits.

Finally, the orthopaedic surgeon decided that I needed an operation that would render me permanently disabled by placing a metal plate on my spine: I would never again be able to ski or dive. It felt wrong; I had no trust in his skills and decided to seek alternative therapy. I found an osteopath who immediately explained that they were treating the symptoms and not the actual cause. He, along with reflexology, reike and massage therapy fixed my back problem. I never looked back. I was one of the most active people I knew. But the fear of disability and losing my health, the vulnerability I felt stayed with me and left me in dread of the day such illness might return.

A twin pregnancy was asking a lot of my back and I worked very hard to do everything I could to keep any problems at bay. My GP referred me to a different physiotherapist and that, along with yoga and walking, kept me going. In fact, women with no back history had more problems than I did. We had the safest twins possible: Dichorionic Diamniotic twins; they each had their own placenta and amniotic sac. It was not possible to tell, during pregnancy, whether they were identical or not. However, since we had IVF it was highly likely that they were dizygotic twins (more commonly referred to as fraternal twins). This meant that they were two eggs fertilised by two sperm. There were twins on my side of the family and the statistics say twins on the woman's side also meant non-identical. It was surprising how many ways twins could form.

Overall, the first trimester was not unpleasant and I marveled at my growing bump, the hormones, the emotions and the miracle of it all. I was reading a lot, being somewhat of an information junkie, and devoured every book I could get hold of. I was somewhat gutted that I couldn't afford to go to spas and have "bump" treatments, I would have loved to pamper myself a little but I knew I could not complain. It was just a shame that our lack of finances was ruining such a beautiful moment. It was hard for me to get used to because I had been used to two large salaries coming in and no longer earned any of our household income. It bothered me more than I realised. I hadn't had to budget since I was a student. I regretted so many things I had purchased before IVF and pregnancy that now seem irrelevant and a waste of money. I should have saved more. I found the animals increasingly clingy and there was a major war going on between my Siamese and moggy cat: they were peeing all over the place. The cats were jealous of my pregnancy. I had to replace a carpet in one bedroom and another on the stairs. This must not continue, I couldn't afford it and needed a clean home for my beloved babies. It seemed to be getting dirtier and more disgusting by the day – they were even pissing on our bed while we were sleeping – I'd never had that happen before! I understood cats didn't like pregnancy and babies but this was ludicrous!

I met Rachel, my midwife and heard their first heartbeats. It sounded like galloping horses and I burst out crying. I saw my obstetrician at seventeen weeks and had an internal scan, the intrusion begins again, to monitor my cervix for premature birth. I learned that I had a very long cervix so was unlikely to be popping them out too early. I wondered if this contributed to us not getting pregnant naturally – an extra long way for his little soldiers, trapped in the surrounding liquid to swim? One twin blew bubbles on the scan as he/she hiccupped and we saw a full face on the screen. I was amazed because I could swear it was like a black and white image of James staring back at me. It was so weird to see a face so clearly. By eighteen weeks I was 13 stone 10 and my bump was 46". I looked about two months more pregnant than I was. I was having my bikini line waxed as I couldn't reach it and this would probably be the last time it got done. My bump was moving all over the place and the young girl waxing me completely freaked out and jumped back when it jolted up like something from *Alien*. I loved watching it every day but James was bored. He occasionally woke up and briefly stroked the bump. I loved lying in the sun and feeling it on my bump wondering how red or dark it must be in there for them. I wondered how these twins would see us and whether it will be in the same way we see ourselves. It scared me that we would be role models for them when we were both so imperfect and had so many things to work on ourselves. Will they see our weaknesses more than our strengths, as we do? Will they spend their lives trying hard to be everything we are not and ensure they don't turn out like us or will they be proud of us and want to adopt our characteristics? It was a daunting prospect becoming a parent. James has been talking about his future plans and all the things we could do as a family to ensure that they had a wonderful childhood. I felt as if I knew them already and as if they had always been here. I often wondered how I would think of them when they were out.

We wanted to surprise ourselves upon birth with regards to their sex but as we walked in to the room for our twenty week scan we both wavered.

"I'm dying to know what sex they are," I said excitedly.

James looked at me. "Me too, I think we should find out."

"Oh no, don't say that, you'll make me weaken and I really want a surprise!"

"Then we won't ask."

"But I want to now that you've said that."

We both smiled. We had spent years moaning about how people didn't value surprise anymore and promised we would never find out in advance only to be fickle and change our minds in an instant. One of them was hiding and we couldn't complete the anomaly scan so had to return a week later. I saw one was definitely a boy, but I was not completely convinced the nurse was right about the other being a girl. One of each sounded perfect. My daughter stayed mostly under my ribs and tries to move around but he doesn't let her – he hogs the exit route. One morning, I was in bed with a cup of tea, taking it easy and reading. Suddenly, my whole bump began to move and little lumps appeared everywhere. It looked like they were having a boxing match in there! I watched, stunned with fascination before I poked the bumps. They went very still for a moment, then bumped back. I poked, they responded and we played for a while like this. It was my first proper interaction with them and I marvelled at how they knew I was there. In yoga they moved constantly and made it hard for me to move from one position to another. I wouldn't get out of bed until we had had our morning play and it was like clockwork just after eight.

At twenty four weeks we opted to pay for a 4D scan and overall we considered it a waste of money unless you had lots to spare. I was surprised how different they looked to each other, even this young, and I wondered if it was a true resemblance. They were very active and wouldn't stop moving so the images weren't great, worse still since they're twins. However, we got a lovely photo of our son smiling and a close up of my daughter looking demur with him sucking his thumb in the background. My pelvis was killing me so the pain took away some of the enjoyment and it was a struggle getting on and off the bed. I hated my younger sister laughing at me, she said I was fat before adding that she was only joking. I had never liked people who used jokes as a way of delivering insults. I despised her immaturity and regretted inviting her to the scan and ruining it since I felt so self-conscious by the end. She was incredibly jealous of me, even more so lately because she believed that I had everything she wanted: marriage, a home and children – she found being single in her thirties very hard. It had always been like this between us. It started with me having large breasts and her having to get a breast enhancement done. She claimed I stole everything first because I was older and first in the queue. My parents caused a lot of sibling jealousy between all five of us with their favouritism. It's draining to be around and maintaining a good relationship was very difficult. I loved her dearly and knew that none of us siblings had been raised to show respect or consideration towards other people but it always ended in someone being offended and I tried to swallow and not bite back but never made it to the end.

While in the bath on a lazy Sunday afternoon, James was poking the bump and laughing as they kicked or punched back. James was excited about becoming a dad. I just wished he would read or sing to them and let them hear his voice. I was really enjoying this pregnancy and was saddened that it was likely to be my only one. I reminded myself that it was better than none. I was also dying to hold them and smother them in kisses. My heart went out to women who never got to where I was – life could be so unfair and hurtful. I wished every woman could feel like I did at that moment. I had never felt this good.

By week twenty six, I weighed 15 stone and my bump was a huge 50.5 inches. I saw the midwife again. My son was horizontal, hip-to-hip and she was breeched with her head rammed under my ribs. Everything was good except my pelvis pain – it was pretty diabolical. I couldn't believe I was a size fourteen on the bottom, sixteen on top because of my enlarged breasts and weighed 15 stone. I really enjoyed this visit because she reassured me and patiently listened to and answered my ridiculous amount of questions. I knew from what other people had told me that I was incredibly lucky to have such a good midwife. She was also very understanding of my pelvis problems and helped me to emotionally handle it by explaining all that my body is going through. I would love her to be a dear friend who I could see all the time – I shall miss her when the twins arrived and wished I could have a home birth in a pool with her – not an option with twins. She was also a breastfeeding specialist and said I could call on her anytime when they were born. She told me to ignore the old fashioned "check for ten movements" everyday, which was a great relief because it was impossible and did nothing but worried me sick.

My son was constantly on the go, it was just my daughter I struggled to feel so I was always relieved when she did something. I worried about how little she moved compared to him. I felt frumpy and hated maternity nightwear and underwear – it was boring and ugly – at least the sort I could afford. Every time I thought of them arriving and getting to hold them I burst out crying. I would miss being pregnant, of this I was certain, I had loved so much of it. I was overpowered by the feelings I had for the twins and how I would do absolutely anything for them. I was overflowing with love, contentment and happiness. Friday morning yoga class was fun and we took turns bringing in tea and cake. Listening to the other girls made me grateful that I didn't have to work and could just take the pregnancy in my stride. I was lucky not having to struggle at work like they were. I was finished between 2 and 4 on the afternoon, as were they, and I could just put my feet up while they struggled through the rest of the day. I was so lucky and grateful. It was great walking Fudge and enjoying the weather. I spent the rest of my time dancing to music and doing chores – my back was bearable – everything was good.

I was really getting into yoga and loved the fact that you could do a workout to recharge you or one to help you sleep. I wished I had found this earlier in my life. I was treating myself to reflexology once a week and that helped with everything, especially the back. I could not be bothered with the online forums, preferring to relish each moment of the day. I loved not being a slave to technology in anyway – no blackberry, mobile etc. I felt so free. I was very aware of how increasingly relaxed I was. I was becoming more separated from the rest of the world. Fudge had an abundance of energy and I was stealing it from her or feeding from it. I loved having a dog. It made such a difference to my daily life and mood. I had completed my birth plan and emailed it to my consultant at the hospital. It must have scared him because he invited me in for a chat. I think he thought I was terrified of it – which was true – and wanted to put my mind at ease but soon realised that I was just really anal. I don't suppose he gets such birth plans often. I was aware that it was too much and too in-depth but couldn't help myself – I had to cover everything. My consultant accepted my birth plan and gave me some crucial advice.

"Your pregnancy is the most important part and avoiding prematurity is key. Don't focus on how they enter this world. How they come out is irrelevant because it becomes obvious through pregnancy what is the safest option so just wait and see. Your yoga is not wasted if you have a caesarean because it will give you a faster recovery. Remember, how they arrive is irrelevant as long as it's safely."

How could I argue with that? Such a patient man, he didn't even blink at the extra sixty questions I handed him to discuss in addition to the birth plan. I was worried but I was also an excited information junkie who wanted to know absolutely everything about this amazing situation I was in. They probably had arguments over which one got to deal with me from then on. It turned out to be the last time I saw him and I felt guilty for taking up so much of his precious time with my trivial fears. I saw the consultant at the hospital, weighing 15.5 stones. It was incredibly hot and I couldn't bear to wear clothes with the heat and size of my bump so I turned up in a sarong and didn't care what I look like – I was a lot more comfortable than the other pregnant women in jeans. I had to pee in a pot, get weighed, walk to the waiting room and sweat for over half an hour after my appointment was due. I saw a student, which didn't please me. I wanted the well-known specialist I was assigned but realised that I was having a healthy pregnancy and he only saw the problem ones. I decided to get over my ego of always wanting the best plus I ignored the fact that I probably scared him away. The twins were doing very well and were close in weight: she was estimated at 3lbs and he was 2lbs 14 oz.

By week 30 frustration was kicking in and I was torn between feelings of hoping I went full term and wanting them out because they were so big I couldn't imagine another eight weeks of growing – how could my body possibly do that? I was gigantic! This had become a massive struggle; I was in agony and movement was limited. I got strangers stare at me in shock because they couldn't believe how big I was and could still walk some even felt the need to comment on how *"I must be about to drop"* – I had ten weeks of such comments to look forward to and it was already tedious and irritating. I was grumpy and unpleasant.

I continued to walk the dog for an hour every day and the other pregnant women could not keep up with me. One walk and they never ask to join me again. The babies were big enough to stroke and hold through the skin now and sometimes it felt as if I was cradling them in my hands. It was easier to stroke my girl because she was so high up, holding the pent-house suite as one nurse said. I could tap her little bottom or stroke her head and it was amazing. I aggravated her with my prodding just to check she was still alive. It was not so cute, however, when she returned to her favourite position and rammed her head right up under my ribcage and gave me the most terrible heartburn for hours at a time rendering me useless for anything until she moved. At least she didn't kick or punch like my son and sometimes I was certain he was going to break out with force. From the earliest of days I could tell them apart by the completely different ways they move. He was the cause of all the pelvis problems because he was so low and he hardly ever stopped moving about. James was the same, kicking and turning all through the night, and now my son strangely did the same. He had powerful kicks! Sometimes they were so sudden and hard they made me gasp and then he would go crazy for a while before settling back down. I was spiritual and natural, which contrasts to my full-on personality and James often laughed at my funny ways and the promises I made on how healthy my children will be.

"Don't blame me if they grow up to be lentil munching tree huggers," he often joked.

He and his family commented on what a proper gentleman's family we were having with a twin son and a daughter in one go, which seemed a strange thing to say to me but he liked the idea, and he was obviously very proud. How different our lives were from only a year ago and how different next year will be. I was a normal person again, treated normally for being pregnant and not avoided for being lost in longing. I could move on with life instead of being in the realms of infertility limbo. I looked forward to our first Christmas together. Until now, Christmases had been a rather sad time for me, always feeling that something was missing. At thirty two weeks I saw the consultant for another brief check up. I was very swollen due to the heat wave we were having (I put my plastic chair in a giant paddling pool and sat in it). They claimed that it wasn't pre-eclampsia. They messed up the scan so we weren't sure of the weights and they were both breech. The level of support was slipping and I was aware that this was because I was low risk and everything was going well. My hope for a drug free natural birth was looking unlikely. A natural birth would help me emotionally by neutralising the clinical and unnatural conception. No one would deliver breech twins naturally – caesarean only. I had to keep my feet elevated for more than 20 hours a day to help reduce the swelling. I had no energy. They were both so active and being breech meant they kicked so hard down below I was certain they would break out. I woke up from nightmares to find a foot, or three, hanging out. I was terrified. I kept puking up unexpectedly and having to quickly swallow it back down before anyone saw – disgusting! My blood pressure was low and yoga was really hard so I started aqua natal instead.

The discomfort was bad and it was horrible not being able to shave, paint your nails, wax, bend, and touch feet. James wouldn't even paint my toe nails for me as some of my friends explained how they had gotten around this problem. He was horribly distant and I felt as if I had been cast out of his life. He had completely withdrawn from me and I missed his company. I felt needy and clingy as I tried to engage him and repeatedly failed. I could never sit, lie or walk comfortably and it was stopping me from getting the rest I needed. I was also bored and starting to realise that friends I thought were close were actually more like acquaintances or I was closer to them than they were to me. Everyone was busy with their fast paced lives and couldn't find the time to visit whereas my days were starting to drag. In fairness, I had always worked long hours too so suddenly expected my friends to change with me. I was becoming more serious too and hoped it was just nerves and worry and I wasn't going to turn into a seriously stressed and miserable mum. I couldn't sleep well, what with the strange dreams and constant peeing and discomfort. To be honest, I felt sorry for myself and I was not proud of that. We spent a day on the beach, since it was so hot, and I swam with the dog. I was too big for a pregnancy costume so instead wore a red bikini top (the only one that fitted) and James's long swim shorts. I looked a huge and shocking sight. It was obvious from the shocked faces and double-takes I got as I walked along the beach, pleased to not have any stretch marks. I felt more beautiful than I looked. At home, I was forced to watch TV on all fours resting on an aerobics ball. Fudge sat beside me sniffing the babies excitedly while Chi Chi, the Siamese, glared at my bump with pure hatred. Sadly, I had to re-home the other cat as they were fighting far too much and costing a fortune in new carpets. The final straw came when she followed me into the toilet and as I sat down she sprayed urine all up my leg. I had never seen a cat do that before and that made the decision I had so far failed to make. I could not have her doing that on my babies. Sadly, she died of leukaemia within a month of being re-homed, which explained the stress and behaviour problems brought out by my pregnancy and left me feeling guilty for not realising she was dying and letting her down. I felt horrible.

  By week thirty four I weighed a massive 16.8 stone and my bump measured 52". I had an unplanned visit to the hospital after a weekend of limited movement – I was adamant I'd lost my little girl. I felt numb and sick. I spent close to three hours being monitored. The tears came and went. I was a wreck – I knew it was all too good to be true. My mind ran riot with all the things that had happened and I was convinced that at least one was being strangled by the umbilical cord. However, everything was fine. Since my son was hogging the best place down below, my little girl was rammed up under my ribs and couldn't move. The nurses were kind and friendly and told me they were not surprised that I had come in: it was next to impossible to monitor movement given the circumstances. I guessed they were just trying to make me feel less embarrassed about wasting their time but I appreciated the kindness. They were heart shaped in my womb: their nose and foreheads touching during the scan – it was beautiful. It was not long after this visit that I began to suspect they wanted out. James kept calling me a bad mum, and he meant it, because I wanted them out and it made me feel guilty. I put the co-sleeper up at the side of our bed ready because I felt the time was close and he made me feel terrible about doing it, refusing to help because I was "forcing them out."

    A local young girl had her baby delivered at home by a friend, she was barely seventeen and laid back about the whole birthing process, this being her second baby, and shared none of my fears. Another lady had her second baby in the garden, with the help of neighbours, and felt no keen desire to get to hospital. It astounded me how different I was because of the infertility and IVF and how precious these little lives are to me. I was overly fearful and protective of my pregnancy. I yearned to feel as relaxed and laid back as those women. However, there were then stories that justified my fears and a young girl in my aqua natal class, in her mid-twenties lost her baby tragically during labour. It was such a freak accident and terribly unfortunate when the umbilical cord caused strangulation. She was younger and fitter than me – there were no guarantees. I was terrified of losing them and heard many sad stories of one or both twins being lost during or soon after birth. In one sense I yearned for the carefree feelings that some women experience and in another I knew the risks were real.

    During yoga, one of the girls brought her new born baby in and when the baby cried my nipples started to produce milk. I started to get really excited, knowing they would be here soon. By week thirty six I weighed seventeen stone. I was really struggling with the weight of my bump and couldn't do anything. Walking up stairs was almost impossible because the bump was huge and low, denying my legs the space to bend. I doubted I would get any stretch marks now – I couldn't believe it – I was so certain I would get "twin skin."   I had drunk lots of water and rubbed in extra virgin olive oil from the second trimester. I loved olive oil. I refused to spend loads of money on creams and it paid off.

***

It was 21:00 and, as usual, I was on the phone all evening. I was mobile enough to walk Fudge daily and prepare food but then lay bedridden for the rest of the day. I was bored and lonely and looked forward to when my friends were home from work on the evenings because James may as well not be here – he was in a permanent sulk – I nicknamed him Victor Meldrew from *One foot in the grave* because he was just like him in character. My bump had dropped and banged off my thighs as I walked slowly and uncomfortably like a whale struggling to prove it could walk on dry land. During my phone call I gasped in pain when my little boy kicked me. It stopped me talking when it happened, it was that strong, but since it was only down below I knew it wasn't a contraction. What didn't occur to me was that I hadn't felt anything above the belly button for weeks. I could watch an arm, an elbow, or a head move the skin on my bump but I couldn't feel it. I just didn't know that you could lose the feeling in part of your bump and then not feel contractions – everyone feels contractions – right? I went to sleep and struggled to get comfortable.

At 02:55 I awoke with the horrible feeling that I was wetting myself but as I became more conscious I realised there was not a bladder in the world that could hold this much pee. I thumped James in the back. He mumbled.

"My waters have broke," I squeaked.

He sat bolt upright, quick as lightening, his back to me. "What do I need to do?"

He was like a robot, alert and attentive but he didn't look at me. I smiled at how odd it seemed. I forced myself to be calm as I realised that I was going to have to do all the directing. I was hoping he might just look after me, he knew the drill, but I could see he needed instructions.

"Get me the phone, first get me towels, grab the bags and load the car – you know the drill."

I had, after all, listed it, printed it, laminated it and made him rehearse it! I called the hospital and they were expecting us. Water poured from me in a way that shocked me – I had never seen so much and couldn't believe it was all coming from me. Thank God I had put that waterproof mattress cover on! Considering how fearful I had been of anything bad happening during labour I became suddenly calm. I couldn't move for ages because the water was still pouring from me. There was no turning back now, not with the waters breaking – this was crunch time. We were in hospital within thirty minutes – James had followed the drill perfectly – I was impressed. We were monitored and held in a room for a while. I was asked if I was sure my waters had broken and she wouldn't take my word for it – had to be shown – which was humiliating and reminded me of my older sister doing the same thing to me when I was twelve and said I'd started my period. However, there were bigger things to think about. I was having contractions that I couldn't feel but I was OK to wait until the morning shift started. I was relieved to do that because I figured it was better to have someone in fresh from a good night's sleep. I decided that the new staff couldn't possibly be hung over from a big night out since it was only mid-week. At the time I didn't realise that my uterus was so extended that I had lost all feeling and that was why I was unaware of the contractions. All I was ever told was that I would know when I was having contractions – it was just as well my waters broke. I was taken into theatre while James was left to get into scrubs. It was nerve racking walking into that theatre and I didn't like the epidural at all – it really hurt. I was terrified by the room. The staff were really good and introduced themselves one at a time, not overwhelming me with the twenty odd staff taking care of me, I never saw more than a couple at a time, it was really well managed.

I did not, however, appreciate the constant referral to my husband being a solicitor and their jokes that they must make sure they didn't make a mistake. It made me feel that their "jokes" was their way of letting me know they felt the need to watch their backs with us and that concerned me: I wanted them to do a good job for me and my babies not because they were scared of getting sued. Not for the first time in my marriage, I wished James had a different profession. Some people despised lawyers and comments were always made to me, never to him. It made me nervous. James robotically walked in and stood beside me, the tears in his eyes choking me up. I had never seen him look like this before. The emotios overwhelmed him. He gently slipped his hand into mine and gave it a squeeze. It was such an emotional moment. They busily worked away behind the curtain.

"Would you like us to lower the curtain and show you the placentas?" we were asked.

"No, we're good thanks," James said with horror-struck eyes.

Then, suddenly, Chris was lifted into the air and began to cry. He was all blue, wriggly and skinny. I couldn't breathe. James was astounded. Immediately afterwards, Beth was lifted up, crying, and she looked so big in comparison.

"Oh my God, she's huge!" James exclaimed.

I finally lost my doubts that I was having two boys and accepted that it was, indeed, one of each. I knew James was tearful as he tried to take photos of them being weighed whereas I was in shock. It felt unreal. Chris weighed 5lb 14 oz and Beth weighed 6lb 9oz. They were good sizes and born barely a minute apart. Their APGAR scores were fantastic: Chris was 9, 10, 10 and Beth was 10, 10, 10. It was hard to put into words the extraordinary emotions that run through you when you see your child for the first time. I felt as if my heart had been ripped wide open with an abundance of love that shook my entire being. They stopped crying as soon as they were handed to me and I hummed to them. My classical music was still playing in the background but I couldn't hear it anymore: my ears buzzed and I was awestruck staring down at these two tiny babies that fascinated me. They struggled to open their eyes and the gunk and bright lights weren't helping. I gently stroked their eyes. Their bodies were quite hairy and Beth's little ears and back were as black as a monkey's - it was adorable. Both had masses of hair; Chris white blonde and Beth dark brown. They were identical to us: Chris was James and Beth was me - we had simply reincarnated ourselves as brother and sister. It was uncanny. The first thing we noticed was her fingernails; she looked like she had a perfect French manicure. There wasn't a spot, blemish, birthmark on either of them – they were impeccably perfect. It suddenly didn't matter to me how clinical their creation or delivery was; they were now just beautiful little miracles. The IVF and misery was long forgotten. I also felt oddly removed from it all, as if I wasn't really there. I wrote the staff a very long, since I was verbose in every way, and thankful letter afterwards because they had done a wonderful job on my caesarean and how they had handled my shyness with so many people was just amazing. I had been told how twenty-two medical staff had stood in a circle around my friend during an unexpected caesarean and it scared her so much she burst out crying. I had expressed my shyness in the birth plan and they had shown immense understanding. It had all progressed perfectly. They had done an amazing, respectful and professional job.

Chapter 5 - Stephen and Claire

Stephen and Claire are tall, dark, slim and attractive. They strike me as the model couple and with their children come across as the perfect family. Claire is sultry, reserved, lady-like and the sort of woman who always seems to be relaxed and in control. I tell myself that she shouts too. She is a strong woman, very organised, determined and keeps herself busy. Stephen, on the other hand, is somewhat mad. He will be the one lying on his stomach on a sleigh with a couple of kids on his back; doing some sort of sport most men twenty years younger lack the stamina for; wearing a sarong in front of "manly-men" and coming off the bigger man despite the teasing. Stephen creates fun from everything he does.

My favourite picture of them, as I always picture them, is as a family, smiling broadly on a small boat. When I look at this family, I see fun...fun...fun... To hear what they have been through you would never imagine it. They have a complicated past, filled with hardship and worry, and have overcome each obstacle without lingering on it. They seem to approach life with the attitude that only today matters and you just have to get on with it. It's an attitude that has paid off.

Lucy, Stephen's first wife, had been complaining about how his life was still fun and that she was always at home having to look after their girls, Emma, aged three, and Hannah aged eighteen months. She wasn't happy. Lucy wanted to move abroad, saying that the UK was no longer a place to bring up a family. Stephen had just been approached by an ex-boss with an opportunity that was perfect for them: a new start up business needing a manager for at least a year in the South of France. It seemed perfect; until the day he was driving home from work, having handed in his notice, to learn via a phone call that Lucy was handing in her notice - on their marriage. She was leaving and going back to a previous relationship. Stephen had no idea what this meant - was he going to lose his two daughters and rarely see them? He was a doting and committed father but had a full time job that could not be done part time. Thoughts raced through his mind as he raced through the traffic. This was not something he had expected to happen.

"You're taking the girls from me?" he asked, dreading the response as he watched her packing her bags.

Lucy looked at him, surprised. "God no! Don't you get it? I don't want to do this: I can't be a mother like this."

"So, you're leaving me with the kids?" he gulped.

Lucy had been a fulltime stay-at-home mum. What would he do with them?

Lucy sighed and rolled her eyes. "I'll take one if you insist but that's all."

Stephen stared at her, shocked, and felt his blood run cold. "I'm not having them split up," he said quietly and with determination. "How do you think they would feel about that?"

"Fine, but I'm still leaving."

They managed to keep things amicable and agreed that Lucy would leave in a couple of weeks once Stephen had managed to arrange some sort of interim childcare. Part of that agreement was to allow Stephen to meet an important commitment attending to a fund raising event at Glastonbury. He was run off his feet and over-committed. Another unexpected phone call ordered him to get home: she was leaving despite the agreement, and had decided she did not want to stay in the house any longer. She left as he came in the door, without a word to the girls. Stephen was barely thirty-three years old and had to remain professional at work while his entire world fell apart. He travelled a lot and that made keeping his two little girls, whose lives had been thrown into disarray - very hard to manage.

So began Stephen's challenging journey down the route of nanny's and au pair's, some good, some wonderful and some *not*! The impact was greater on the older daughter and her behaviour was, understandably, difficult. They were fine with the first nanny partly because they were so young and in their minds at least mummy would be coming back: as Lucy would tell them. After the second nanny, which was a traumatic experience for all, they became harder to look after and saw a few childminders away. One day, while the girls were being very difficult, the new au pair cracked and called Stephen at work. He was in a meeting. Unable to contact him, the au pair called Lucy, who came over and watched the children with the au pair until Stephen returned. Stephen was not best pleased; the girls had learned that if they behaved badly they would get their mother back. In addition, she undermined the au pair and walked away leaving a very difficult situation to work through.

One of Stephen's friends, who he occasionally does sport with, had a lovely wife, who had a lovely sister: Claire. They conspired to bring the two of them together. The four of them went to a Paul McKenna event but nothing exciting happened, other than the show. Then they met again on another weekend away, once more nothing special occurred. On the third attempt to matchmake they went on a boat trip with a small group of people - that was when they clicked. The reason nothing happened the first two times was because Stephen really didn't want a relationship – he was done with women – but Claire won him over and he fell for her. She was seven years younger, knew how to handle him, and fitted in perfectly with his life: she didn't want children. Stephen just wanted to have some fun now that his girls were getting older.

Emma was eight and Hannah was six when Claire first met them at Stephen's home. She was petrified: the girls were very confident and were used to different people coming and going in their house whereas Claire was quiet and reserved with absolutely no experience of children. Fortunately, they were very affectionate and full of life and energy and soon made her feel comfortable. Only that first half hour was scary for Claire and after that she just clicked with the girls. They put on a show for her, some singing and dancing, and she loved them straight away. Claire had two Springer spaniels and when the girls met them it was love all around. They were together for twenty months before they sold their homes and moved in together. It was the second time around for both of them and they knew what they were doing and that they worked well together. It was perfect – for a while.

Stephen thinks that raising his two girls from the ages of six and eight started Claire's body clock ticking and changed her mind about wanting her own children, but Claire doesn't agree. Something big had changed: she now wanted children. Stephen was adamant that he didn't and that this was his time to start living life to the full, his life had been hard, but his love for Claire soon overruled and he gave in.

"I warned her," he explains, "that it would rock our world and change our lives completely. She had no experience of young children, mine were older when she started to raise them and it's a whole different kettle of fish when they're really young. I felt as if I had only just got my freedom back. We had some tearful arguments about it and she told me that if I wouldn't let her have children then I wasn't the right man for her. A good friend of mine gave me some invaluable advice: if you really love each other, and she desperately wants children, then there is only one thing to do. He was right. I could not deny her the children that she craved."

They tried for a year to get pregnant. Claire was thirty eight, Stephen was forty five. They were referred to the hospital for tests. Apart from blood tests, they had a post-coital examination done, which checks the woman's cervical mucus after sex to see whether the sperm is still present and moving. There wasn't a clear problem with the cervical mucus; it may have been slightly acidic, resulting in Stephen's sperm struggling to move. Then, she had the laparoscopy and dye test, that was not supposed to hurt, and Claire was in unexpected agony. Her sister had been through this and hadn't felt a thing. Another woman returned to the hospital while Claire was still there and had to be given morphine. Claire didn't have morphine but was disappointed that she wasn't warned that it could hurt so much. They were put on clomid and had more post-coital tests. Stephen wasn't excited about Claire being on clomid because he was very worried about multiple births, something he didn't like the risks of and disliked anything unnatural.

"I hated this," Stephen sighs. "And the sex on demand was really difficult because I preferred us both to enjoy sex and have orgasms which is hard under these circumstances. It was very clinical and mechanical and Claire was so frustrated that she couldn't relax. It was not a nice thing to have to do."

After one month, Claire had a positive pregnancy test. At a seven week scan she was told that it was not a viable pregnancy, there was nothing but a sac, and it didn't look good. It was gut-wrenching for them both. They had even told people that they were pregnant. Claire held her breath and hoped that the scan was wrong. At a ten week scan she was told the same thing. They offered her a D&C, she refused, innocently hoping that she might be giving her baby the chance to revive itself and come back somehow. She was in denial until she had a natural miscarriage which hurt her immensely and brought her cruelly back to reality. Further tests revealed that Claire was showing signs of the menopause so they decided to go for IVF. Claire was really excited about this: she had a goal and just wanted to achieve it. Stephen, however, was in a difficult position: he did not believe in IVF. He felt that science was going against natural selection and messing with the human gene pool; babies are being kept alive from twenty four weeks; old people forced to battle on longer than their bodies can cope; even caesarean sections do not sit well with Stephen. It put him in a difficult situation.

Claire began taking the drugs with rapture. Terrified of not taking the drugs at the correct time she hid a timer down her cleavage. The needles terrified her and they had chosen a supplier who provided them with smaller needles, for a slightly higher price, which she happily paid. She found them easier than expected. Due to the tests suggesting she was nearing menopause, they had given her a higher dosage of drugs and she soon became over stimulated. It was too dangerous to remove her eggs and they abandoned the cycle, losing all the money, everything an utter waste of time. They were mortified but accepted that they knew this could happen. They stood up for round two.

Stephen wasn't impressed with his part of the process. "It was bloody awkward having to produce on demand," he exclaims with passion. "I could have done with some help! Unfortunately, the room and the material given were bland in the extreme."

"Did they not ask if you wanted Claire to go in or if you wanted to freeze a sample in advance, just in case? They asked me and James."

"That would have been perfect but they didn't suggest that as a possibility. It was hard work trying to aim into those silly little pots. Bloody difficult and very awkward!"

The next round of IVF was successful and they retrieved ten eggs. Six fertilised naturally but when it came to implantation only two were good enough to use. In early December they were both implanted and the wait for the pregnancy test began: this would be a very happy or a sad Christmas. The day of the test arrived and it was positive. They were ecstatic. Then, barely four days later, she had a massive bleed. Trying to contain their emotions they went for a scan. It was not a viable pregnancy and they were advised to just continue doing pregnancy tests until they went back to negative and then they would see her again. With each pregnancy test the line faded, dampening her hopes, until one day it was stronger. Claire grew excited – perhaps she had only lost one of the embryos? Two days before Christmas she was told that she might have an ectopic pregnancy. On Boxing day, her hormone levels had increased.

"I kept thinking: come on, I know you're in there somewhere!" Claire says.

She had a laparoscopy and was warned beforehand that they might have to remove a tube or, the worst case scenario, do an entire hysterectomy there and then. They knew that the staff were legally obliged to warn them of these things, and that is was not likely, but this didn't make the fact that it could happen any less worrying. Fortunately, they couldn't find anything and told her it might be in her abdomen somewhere - there might still be hope. But with each pregnancy test the line faded and her hormone levels, being closely monitored, began to come down. In January, a month after her first miscarriage, she had another big bleed and that was the end of the pregnancy. Stephen and Claire, being who they are, brushed themselves off and went for round three: and completely messed it up right at the beginning.

"We were going skiing and I completely forgot about the drugs!" Claire says. "I had to ask my sister to collect them, since there was no time to allow for postage, which meant telling her what was going on, which we'd kept a secret after that first awkward time of telling people. I opened the drugs on the plane and to my horror I realised that not all the drugs were in the packet! There was a prescription. We had to find a pharmacist in Italy and were really worried that we weren't going to be able to do this but he was wonderful and told us to leave it with him. Mercifully, he came through."

This time they had eight eggs and four or five fertilised, as she tries to recall. However, she does remember that once more only two were good enough.

"When I did the test," she says, pausing for a moment as she chokes up and is unable to speak, "it was again positive but this time I felt much more confident and I knew I was pregnant and that everything would be OK. I had sore boobs too, which I hadn't had before and somehow I just knew this was OK."

She cried when they saw the heartbeat on the scan and was told that there was a 98% chance of having a live birth. This lifted Claire's spirits tremendously and she beamed with joy.

"I had a good pregnancy and was only a little nauseous: smells bothered me immensely, especially wet dog and buttercups. I couldn't stand the smell of buttercups and if the dogs went into a buttercup field I was gagging – it was vile. I remember the smells!"

They tried to keep it secret and told one set of friends that they weren't going to see for a while. Shortly thereafter, they received a congratulations card from them that was seen by other visitors to the house - the cat was out of the bag.

"I insisted on all the tests," Stephen says.

"Yes, that's one thing Stephen was very particular about," she admits. "He wouldn't consider having a child with anything wrong with it. This was the hardest thing for me to emotionally face. The risk of miscarriage with the tests was terrifying and I couldn't stop crying, I got myself very worked up. I didn't know what I would do if the results were bad. We paid for them to come through quicker and they were good. I was then able to relax and enjoy the pregnancy, telling everyone that it was all fine. I had a great pregnancy then, after those first fifteen weeks, despite the swollen ankles and carpel tunnel."

At their twenty week scan the baby was showing a low-lying placenta so she was closely monitored for needing a caesarean and had several scans due to her age. She chose to schedule in a caesarean when the time was right, since that seemed the safest route, and was petrified on the morning. She had a spinal block and lay in excitement as they rummaged about to get the baby.

"The caesarean was peculiar - it was like they were rummaging about in a suitcase," Stephen says. "Then out came Alison. It was wonderful."

"I was just so excited at seeing her and impatiently waited for her to appear. Stephen was busy trying to peer over the curtain and see what was happening and as she came out gunk flew all over my chest. The nurse was busy taking loads of shots of her coming out and then they took her away to be cleaned up. I was panicking a little, until I heard her cry and then desperately wanted to hold her and have skin-to-skin contact: I was worried the caesarean would interfere with bonding. But then Stephen took her out and left me there for what seemed like ages to get stitched back up. I don't know why I wasn't given her to hold but when it was over I was breastfeeding her straight away, it only took about fifteen minutes, it was easy. It was sore at first and it hurt but we soon got past that and I really liked it."

Alison was two weeks early and weighed 7 lbs 12 oz. She was a healthy little girl from the start.

"I don't remember much more except the journey home. Claire was cradling Alison in her arms and looked so happy and content and I'll never forget that - it was worth every minute. I have never been happier," Stephen explains.

"I love being a mother. During that awful time of wanting children I would be driving home from work and ponder on what would happen if I couldn't. I was fearful of the prospect of never having a child, and felt so lost and empty, to the point that I even doubted life would be worth living. I burst out crying on many car journeys," Claire explains.

It took them three years to get Alison. When Alison was a year old, and they had been considering another round of IVF for the second child that they wanted, Claire fell pregnant naturally. Like so many women she did the pregnancy test on the day her period was due and the line was so faint that she had doubts. She didn't feel pregnant this time. Upon speaking with her midwife, and fear of an ectopic pregnancy and another miscarriage, they scheduled her in for an early scan.

"I was convinced it wasn't a real pregnancy again," Claire says. "It felt the same as before."

Claire went to the scan alone, knowing what to expect and not feeling the need for Stephen to be there to share the bad news. Stephen went to work as normal. When she called him after the scan she couldn't speak for all the tears and sobbed down the line.

"It's going to be OK," Stephen tells her, having also expected the bad news. "I'm so sorry I'm not there to give you a cuddle, I thought you'd be OK."

"No, it's real. I'm pregnant," she eventually managed to say between sobs.

This time, Claire has no nausea but is really big and incredibly tired. Having Alison running around meant that she couldn't take any naps and the tiredness set in. This time, she chose a natural birth, since the position of the baby was good, and was terrified when her waters broke. There was no sign of the baby coming and they had to induce her. It was scary. She had to remain still, not allowed to move around, as she was tied up to several monitors because of her previous caesarean – she felt tied down and restricted. There was only one other woman in labour so she received ample attention. Within ten minutes of being put on the drip, her contractions began in force. After an eight hour labour, an epidural and six days late, Elly was born weighing 9 lbs 12oz.

Breastfeeding was once more quickly established. Claire had to have stitches and work hard at her pelvic floor exercises.

"I love being a mum and enjoyed breastfeeding them both for about ten months before I'd had enough and wanted my breasts back," Claire says happily. "But it's a lot harder than I thought and the commitment is not what I expected. I never really gave it much thought, I just felt how much I wanted a baby but not really what it meant. The tiredness is constant and I have no energy at all. Sometimes, when I'm really struggling, I don't tell Stephen and ask him for help because I know how much he wants his freedom and didn't want to go through all this again so I feel as if I have to be careful. This was what I wanted. I know he's happy and loves us all but he still needs to feel as if he is getting some freedom back in life. I just feel constantly tired. I don't know what I would do if I only had one because they play so nicely together and I couldn't sit down and entertain just one all the time. I can cook with them and do active things but I can't sit down and do imaginary play so it's nice that they have each other."

Alison is five and Elly three now. They are just coming out of the hardest period and will soon have more freedom. The older girls have little to do with their biological mother, from their own choosing, consider Claire as more of a mother than their biological one and are happy with their new little sisters.

"Looking back, IVF wasn't really that bad," Claire recalls. "I'm glad I did it and have two beautiful children as a result because I wouldn't have Elly if the fertility drugs hadn't kicked my body into gear. I didn't get any pressure from anyone about my age and not yet having kids, probably because I was strongly against having them when I was younger, and my mother never questioned us with anything, she just waited for us all to do whatever we wanted with our lives. I'd recommend IVF to anyone. I feel so fulfilled. There is this wonderful feeling of unconditional love that I have for them and that they have for me. At the time, I was disappointed that we had no viable eggs to freeze but now I'm glad. Since Elly was natural she perhaps wouldn't be here if I had frozen embryos to use. I have a friend who is in a terrible dilemma at the moment: she hit the menopause at thirty and had to have IVF with donor eggs. They had two embryos put in and one frozen; it failed so they had the frozen one put in and had a girl. They did another round of IVF for a second child and had twin boys. They still have two frozen embryos but she is forty seven now and is not in great physical shape. However, there is potential life there with her frozen embryos and she wants to proceed but her husband doesn't because of their age and having three kids already – she just cannot bear to let them go. It's difficult and very emotional. I'm so glad I don't have to face a decision like that."

Claire's worry will never end now that she is a mum and she admits this as she recalls how Elly recently fell off one of those basket swings at the park.

"It was horrifying. There were a few children sitting on the edge of one of those large basket swings, as they had done many times before, and Elly somehow fell off. I don't know how it happened and seeing my perfect little princess broken on the floor and in so much pain was more than I could bear. How dare she be hurt and what a terrible mother I am! I must be a better mother from now on and pay more attention. The two days after were worse because she was in so much discomfort and I could do very little about it. I found it very hard to deal with emotionally."

Stephen is probably less content but only because he doesn't have the same life that he and Claire had shared before, which had been lovely as far as their spark and love life was concerned, he misses that. He adores the children that they have.

"I almost consider myself redundant now," he sighs. "Sometimes I feel I'm no longer needed for sex and, before that, for over a year, it felt clinical and mechanical, so it feels odd now and sometimes I think our sex life has gone."

Claire doesn't share this view and thinks the sex life would be great if only she weren't so exhausted all the time but she does agree that Stephen initiates it nowadays. She is certain that her energy levels will soon return and things will improve. Claire may well be right as they recently celebrated their tenth wedding anniversary and seventeen years together, returning to their honeymoon location and having a passionate time together. It was fantastic – I am reliably informed.

Chapter 6 - The Art Of Blundering Breastfeeding

Our immediate priority, as with all new parents, was to feed them but breastfeeding didn't come naturally to me. They both cried inconsolably. I was unable to hold both of them at the same time and desperately alternated between the two – achieving nothing. Other crying babies on the ward woke them up as much as they woke each other. None of us could sleep. I changed their nappies, tried to feed them, walked them about, despite the caesarean, and kissed them – nothing worked. At five o'clock the next morning, having not slept at all, I look around for help and that was when it hit me: the cold hard reality that I had no one to turn to. It was me they needed and I had to do my best for them both at the same time. It took the wind out of my sails and I felt as if I had been punched. Terror and reality overwhelmed me and I burst into tears. It wasn't possible to look after them both together. They each deserved my undivided attention, like the other babies on the ward were getting, and deserved better than I could provide. I didn't get to sleep until midday – twenty eight hours after my caesarean. When talking to other new mothers in the ward I realised that I had not been thinking normally like they had throughout pregnancy. They, having faced no years of infertility or IVF, had normal thoughts of excitement, parenting, shock, panic and love. Whereas I had been blindly focused on getting pregnant and once that was achieved fearfully ensuring I didn't lose what I had worked so hard to get. I never really thought much about what it would mean being a mother and two babies at once was simply overwhelming.

My blood pressure was sky high and severe pre-eclampsia hit me, which I had thought was only a pregnancy illness. I was scaring the staff. James was told he had to sleep on the floor for seven nights to keep an eye on me; I was not to be left unobserved for a moment because they were scared I would have a stroke or vital organ failure. There was not enough staff to monitor me and the twins. We were warned how serious this was and learned that a woman had died the previous week of the same thing leaving her baby boy alone with his father. The midwife made it clear that my vitals were far worse than the woman who had just died. It shocked me. I watched my twins with fear that I might die, terrified that I had only gone through all this to miss out on their upbringing and leave them with no mother.

I lost almost three stones immediately with the Caesarean. I had a massive stomach but no time to think about it because I was lost in the world of breastfeeding. I had two massive boobs and two tiny heads to work with. I was suddenly being weighted down by two 36J giant cupcakes (I had been a size 36D) with mini-marshmallows for nipples. I couldn't see what I was doing. It perplexed me how a woman's body could get something so basic so wrong – my big breasts did not suit such small babies. The staff were utterly useless. They tried ramming their heads onto my breast, in what seemed a cruel manner that obviously upset the babies and even made Beth turn away from my breast from then on. They groped and squeezed my nipples ineffectively, like I was a piece of meat, and made me wonder how on earth they could be considered midwives. Chris was easier and could suck a little but I was getting nowhere with Beth. They both developed jaundice and we were being pushed to formula feed. I was adamant I didn't want to, having been told to "stick to my guns," and they made me feel terrible about it, accusing me of putting the twin's lives in danger. I started to panic and all my confidence left me. In the space of two days I felt as if I was completely incompetent. They had no time for explanations and rushed in and out.

The jaundice made them too weak to suck and now they were drastically losing weight. I had to formula feed. James did all the bottle feeds since I expressed like a mad woman – every two hours without a break, day and night. I gave every drop of milk I could squeeze out to them and was over the moon when my milk came through. They had formula for a day and a half before I could match their needs with my milk. I knew that I needed expert help to get breastfeeding so accepted bottles while we were in hospital. As I expressed with the double breast pump, I balanced the mobile between my shoulder and chin, and organised professional backup. I ordered a double breastfeeding pump, at £40 a month, to be delivered and arranged for two midwives to visit me when I would be at home. I had learned so much from the LLL (la leche league).

At least the twins were getting my milk for now and all the colostrum. It was all I could do. Neither of us slept for those seven days for more than an hour at a time but adrenaline kept us going. They kept coming in and taking my blood pressure and doping me up with pills they swore were safe while breastfeeding. I hated it but my blood pressure was frighteningly high. Day and night they checked me every couple of hours. I knew they were trying to look after me but a good night's sleep would have been much better. Every time I asked them to let me sleep for a few hours they agreed but then changed shift and a new person would take over and wake me up to check I was still alive. It was ridiculous. I had heard of staff letting the new mothers sleep so failed to understand why they refused to let me sleep considering I was severely ill. It didn't make sense.

They were also taking blood samples from the twin's feet at a rate that horrified me and made them scream in pain, which I couldn't bear, as they monitored their jaundice. Their tiny feet were black and blue. Chris was handling it well but Beth had to go under a heat lamp for treatment for three days. I was terrified of losing her. She didn't look well and I couldn't hold her much during this time. However, hearing much more tragic stories while pumping my milk in the breastfeeding room, about women who had children in intensive care, made me realise how trivial this was. One lady had even been told not to expect to leave the hospital with her baby, that he would undoubtedly die, but she sat there, hour after hour, alongside me pumping out 5 or 10 ml of milk to feed him via tubes for all her life was worth. She was older than me and I couldn't help but wonder what she might have been through to actually get this little boy in the first place – had she faced IVF too? It was a chilling and sobering thought. It still makes me cry thinking about her and I dearly hope she took that little boy home despite the odds and what the doctors said.

The room we were in was fine for a single bed but not all of us, especially with Beth's heat lamp. It was horribly hot, even with the window open the couple of inches it would go. I felt stifled and claustrophobic. I wore a light sarong but still sweated like a pig and looked like one with all my extra weight and the double breast pump attached. I avoided mirrors. We stopped visitors coming when Beth was put under the lamp because we were too emotional and there was little room. I was crying non-stop and almost discharged myself because I knew their poor treatment and the lack of sleep was making me a lot worse. However, with the jaundice I had no choice but to stay. We took a bath towards the end of the week – our first wash. It was a small bath and awkward to manage all four of us. James got in and I passed him one baby at a time. They were called baby boy and baby girl by the nurses and we adopted this, despite having named them during pregnancy, because we thought it cute. "Come, baby boy. Hush, baby girl." We loved saying it. They stopped crying in the water and were all quiet and content afterwards. By the time I got in the water was filthy but I was in no fit state to bend and run a fresh one and it never occurred to James to do it or me to ask him. There wasn't a shower anywhere. I was malodorous.

 I desperately wanted to go home but still they refused to discharge us once the jaundice was better because of my health. The amount of formula our paediatrician expected us to get down each child was unreasonable and impossible – and I felt we were force feeding them. I cried and pleaded, saying it wasn't right and was upsetting them, but I was treated like an idiot and told we couldn't leave until we could prove ourselves capable of getting the required amounts down them. They were so condescending. Even the midwives couldn't get them to take the amounts the paediatrician had told us to give. I later learned that you need less breast milk than formula and should calculate it accordingly. We really had been force feeding them. I hated the place, I hated the staff and I wanted to go home. They were short staffed, had closed down several wards and an entire floor, and were overrun with a baby boom. As a result, they were working under awful conditions and it made them nasty and cynical – not what I needed to be around. They stripped me of my confidence and I was about to learn that it would take me more than two years to get it back again.

 For some bizarre reason, whenever James changed a nappy he mostly got pee'd or pooped on. I never did. It was something about him and it reminded me of how the animals treated him. That was the only thing that made us laugh during the entire week.

I forced the food down me to keep my milk supply going. I always ate it cold and had to yell at the canteen staff not to take it away as I hadn't gotten around to eating it – they really were annoyed by the inconvenience. I often ordered an extra plate because I was breastfeeding twins and needed fuel but they thought I was feeding James for free and refused to provide it. James had to go out and buy me food daily. He lived on sandwiches from the shop. I could have throttled the canteen manager with my bare hands if I hadn't been so busy expressing milk. I was obsessed with needing more milk. If James hadn't been a solicitor, which they still repeatedly mentioned, they wouldn't have been so back-protecting and cold towards us, fearing being sued over and above our welfare. If I hadn't been so high-risk we could have had a nice family room instead of the small one with the beds on wheels. We were, thankfully, distracted by the twin's non-stop nappy changes, feeding, farting and burping. How could babies be so loud? My blood pressure and urich acid remained dangerously high. They wanted to keep me in longer than seven nights, which put me in floods of tears. The jaundice had gone, the children were fine: I remained the problem. I called my GP and begged her help. She and my midwife told the hospital to let us go home, they could support me. We were finally given the all clear at 8:30 PM, which seemed a ridiculous time to me because we could have gone home earlier, had a nice bath and got a good night's sleep at last.

We drove slowly and the twins looked far too small to be in their car seats. My floppy stomach made moving difficult and it had to be carried in my arms. When we got home, at 21:30, my parents-in-law greeted us with Fudge who I hadn't seen since my waters broke. We walked in and James had both the twins in his arms. Fudge sniffed my belly, as she had done for the last eight months, then sniffed the twins and left my belly alone from that day on - she knew. And from that moment she sat near them and guarded them like a little angel. I couldn't have wished for a lovelier dog. The twins settled down well but then woke up in the middle of the night and screamed the place down – they did not like their new cot at the side of my bed – it was bigger than the hospital ones. On top of that, their cries freaked out the Siamese who yowled alongside them, hysterically, which made them scream even more and not one of them would quit. James and I stared at each other in utter shock. It was like triplets but one was furry. That was the moment I lost a lot of my love for that cat and I don't know how I didn't kill her. She came in yowling often, waking them up at four or five in the morning and all hell would break loose again. She learned that I would ignore her yowls for food but if she woke the twins up it would get me out of bed. This beautiful Siamese, who had been my darling baby for seven years, became my nemesis.

Within three days of being home my health improved and the sun was keeping the twins jaundice at bay. My GP and midwife were more concerned about long term damage to my internal organs and I tried not to worry about it. We knew that it would be hard work but we really had no idea what hard work actually meant until we were thrust into the chaos of it all. We were both professionals who worked sixty to eighty hours a week but nothing had been so demanding, relentless and exhausting. On top of sleep deprivation we were defeated. We slept, as best we could, with a baby each on our chests for the first month – it was the only way we could close our eyes. Even then, we didn't really sleep because we were terrified of squashing or dropping them. I was frantically trying to keep up with all their demands. It was overwhelming for both of us and I was getting no time to recover. No one was around to let us sleep for a few hours because no one would have the twins. Even though I was up with them in the night, James could still hear them. My younger sister, who had never been good with animals or children, refused to hold them for the first three months because they looked "too small and might break."

"Can we talk about something other than breastfeeding? I have no interest in it or how hard it is for you, moving on—" she would say with the flat hand gesture I loathed.

I stared blankly at the wall willing my mind to find something else to talk about – I had nothing. She asked if I'd watched Judge Judy, Big Brother or the X factor and cannot believe me when I say I had no time for TV. I decided to just listen about her colleagues, boss and shoddy work environment, which I equally had no interest in, which was OK because I was unable to retain any information. My brain was blank. Even James and his parents were too terrified to even try and have the twins together, as a team, so I could get two or three hours sleep. I always had to be there holding one and the pressure weighed heavily upon my shoulders. I was dropping. My midwife told James he would kill me if he didn't let me get some rest and my blood pressure was still extremely high. I begged and would have done anything for just two hours sleep. Everyone was happy to keep one baby occupied for two or three hours while you rest but twins were harder. The twins club had warned me that grandparents often wouldn't help with multiples. I wanted the twin's father and grandparents to step up to the mark and handle it – not run. The family did what they could and brought us food, did the ironing and tidied up, which helped James, who was doing the cooking and cleaning, but didn't get me the much needed rest or wash I craved. I was ungrateful because all I needed was sleep and recovery and cared little for creases in clothes. It was made very clear that they were here to help James only and not me.

The two midwives came and helped me to breastfeed but it was a battle. Within the first week of being home I had Chris easily on my breast. Nothing worked with Beth. On the third week my midwife realised that she had tongue tie. I went to a breastfeeding clinic and they scheduled her in for a tongue-tie 'snip'. I was a bag of nerves. They were to slice the piece of flesh under her tongue. In the olden days a midwife used to do it with a fingernail kept especially sharp for the purpose. There was blood everywhere - I cried like a baby - Beth didn't blink. Within a week she was breastfeeding and I was finally able to stop expressing – seven weeks to get them both on the breast – I was exhausted. I had a ridiculously fast letdown that gushed out and it was more than Beth could handle: she bit down and frequently blocked my milk ducts.

I attended the breastfeeding clinic regularly, working on perfecting our technique. Beth, during a feed, kicked my spare breast out of her way, sending milk across the room and drenching the outer-thigh of a woman four seats away. Everyone stared in shock. Most of them were there to build up their milk supply and here I was showering them in it! I was so embarrassed and she looked at me with the utmost disgust as she tried to rub it off, only succeeding in rubbing it further in. She never acknowledged my humble apology. The nurse was in stitches on the floor, which broke the ice a little. My breasts were producing far too much milk, because of the double breast pump stimulation, and I donated copious amounts to the intensive care unit at the hospital for the first four months. I had blocked milk ducts and mastitis because of Beth and if she had been my only baby I would have given up. On the other hand, Chris was king of breastfeeding and if Beth "broke" a breast he "fixed" it. They complimented and supported each other right from the start. I envied how mums with one baby could give a sore breast a rest. This was my first experience of singleton envy.

They both had colic and sleep-deprivation was playing with my mind and making me delirious. I didn't know what was a dream and what was real. One night I dragged myself out of bed to feed Chris. I really didn't want to and could have left him to starve but something in me couldn't ignore him. I took him into the nursery and sat on the rocking chair. They were still, at this point, in a co-sleeper next to my bed but I didn't want to wake Beth and James. It killed me staying awake and my head kept dropping – I almost dropped him twice - jolting myself upright just in time. My heart raced and I tried desperately to stay awake and finish the one hour feed. I should have put the futon down in the spare bedroom and lay with him but there was no such thing as common sense in my head at this point in time – I was too exhausted to think straight. With a sigh of relief he finished and dropped away from my breast. I was just pulling up my top when I heard Beth stir.

"You have to be kidding me?" I gasped, looking at the clock. 4:05 AM. I had last fed her two hours ago.

"I can't do it, I just can't do it," I sobbed, burying my head into Chris.

I loathed the feeling of not being able to feed my babies. I seemed useless at doing it from the moment they were born.

I couldn't carry Chris back to bed and spend an hour feeding Beth. They always fed slower at night because they were half asleep. I felt utterly hopeless. James walked in with Beth in his arms.

"Grace, didn't you hear her, she's hungry," he said crossly before realising I was sobbing. "Come on, get to bed, I'll hold her by you while you sleep."

I really was struggling.

I find it hard to care about my body and have no time for it – no time for me. To begin with I was washing with wet wipes – no one would be left with the twins for five minutes – still only holding one while I had the other. I saw other dad's out with their twins so that the wife could sleep. I resented James. I tried to have a bath once; one twin was asleep upstairs and the other downstairs. I dived in the bath and within seven minutes one had woken up. I could hear my mother-in-law getting stressed and trying to settle the baby. Then, for some bizarre reason, she brought the screaming baby upstairs so she could check on the other one, who promptly woke up with all the noise. She barged into the bathroom and threw a baby at me. I was naked and embarrassed and sat holding the baby in a very hot, deep bath, unable to get out because of my stitches. I hadn't even had ten minutes, didn't get to use soap or wet my hair. She just didn't seem to want to even try and let them cry for a few minutes until I got out. It wasn't the first time she barged in on me while I was naked, or almost naked. She did it often while I was expressing. I was so self-conscious of how fat I was, how hideously large my breasts were, and didn't want anyone seeing me like that. Being ignored, upon informing her that it made me feel uncomfortable, bothered me even more.

I was feeding about four babies with the additional milk I was expressing for the hospital. Winding them was hard; their wind got trapped and trying to do both of them at the same time was impossible. There was never enough time to feed and wind one because the other one turned blue screaming for their food. I had an aerobics ball, a large one, and sat on that in the lounge with a baby on each arm and bounced for ages. It worked. I paid £70 for a twins breastfeeding cushion that acted as nothing more than a convenient way of holding them both because I couldn't, for the life of me, tandem feed. James and I were so tired we couldn't hold a civil conversation. My mother-in-law was very helpful and came most days during the first six weeks. Her help getting me to the breastfeeding clinic saved me many bus journeys. She was trying to do her best for the grandchildren. You would have thought we were really good friends. I think she even started to like me a little. I forgave her for how she had treated me in the past and tried to be the daughter-in-law she wanted.

When she went to France, where they part retired, for a few weeks something changed. I didn't know what or why and the only thing I could think of was that we didn't install and set up skype so they could see the babies, as they had asked. However, when James came home from work we faced two hours of manic activity and I went to bed with the twins. They were two months old. We weren't sleeping, struggled through each day and I had no time alone during the day to install and get it working and breastfeeding still took up my entire resources. James spent every evening cleaning up and preparing food for me for the following day – I was unable to eat anything other than junk if he didn't; there was no time to make food while alone with the twins. It was chaos. I think she was just resentful that she had spent so much time with us during those first six weeks and was furious that she had to wait until returning to the UK to see them. We tried to find the time to set up skype but the days just flew by in a blur.

Upon her return, I found her unexpectedly cold and distant and I felt rejected. It hurt because I thought we had found a good relationship in those early weeks. I did not like to be treated in such a fickle way and liked to know where I stood with people. It reminded me of Ben Stiller in 'Meet The Fockers' – desperately trying to gain the parent-in-laws acceptance and the harder I tried the more I screwed up. I often said and did the wrong thing, no matter how hard I tried, it always came out wrong or was taken in the worse possible context. It was almost as comical as the movie; whatever I said was inappropriate and met with disapproval but there was nothing wrong if someone else said or did the same thing. This often made me more awkward and more likely to say or do something inappropriate. As a result, her visits became difficult and I felt that she was only coming to put me down and two full days in a row was full on. James and I constantly rowed over her. I did not want her here – she was making me feel terrible about myself and I wasn't strong enough to cope with her. As usual, he did nothing.

Something dramatic happened at the three month mark. The colic disappeared overnight and I learned to tandem feed. I preferred feeding them one at a time and they now fed quickly. Tandem feeding made me feel like a piece of meat and I only did it to avoid a meltdown which made life much easier. I felt constantly guilty - I manipulated science to have them and now I couldn't look after them. As far as breastfeeding was concerned, for the first time in my life, I felt truly connected with the woman within me and it felt amazing. I was able to just enjoy those relaxing and wonderful breastfeeding hormones and I was in heaven. It was the most amazing experience of my life and I relished it. Things were slowly starting to turn around.

The reason I persevered with breastfeeding far longer than what was healthy for me was because I had a huge issue with the lack of "nature" involved in the conception and birth of my twins. Breastfeeding was the only thing I could give them naturally: I had "failed" to conceive them naturally; "failed" at natural childbirth; and there was no way on earth I was going to "fail" at breastfeeding. If I had watched any of my friends do what I did I would have made them stop and not be so daft. However, in the long run, being able to breastfeed them and enjoy it was priceless. I knew numerous friends and family who couldn't breastfeed or didn't want to for one reason or another and I have no qualms about that. I think it's the best start to give your child but you need to be happy, as does your baby, above all else.

I have a lovely group of new friends the Health Visitor put me in touch with and Tuesday morning was my favourite day of the week; we took our babies to music group then went to a local pub for coffee and cake. In my "mummies group" we were open minded and accepted anyone with any approach to feeding, routine or weaning and I completely believe if it was right for them then it was right – full stop. It was very hard to breastfeed discretely when you had twins and a large pair of breasts: I was annoyed at disapproving glances and comments I occasionally received and became even more self-conscious. Whenever I fed, the twin not being fed screamed and drew attention, if I tandem fed I was virtually topless. Either way, I drew attention. I never expected disapproving looks or comments because I was breastfeeding and it shattered my confidence further. My mother-in-law and sister thought it was disgusting to breastfeed in a restaurant and that it was more acceptable for me to do it in the toilet. Therefore, I felt intimidated and hardly went out in public. We were no longer invited anywhere. We were stressed, the twins prevented us from participating in conversations and we were not great company. Fortunately, it was a warm summer and I spent most of my day breastfeeding in peace along the river as Fudge played in the water. I loved my dog dearly.

    I wanted to breastfeed until they were eighteen months to two years, especially once I was really into it and enjoying it. I watched the hard work other mums had with sterilising bottles, preparing formula and considered it crazy. I found it so much easier to get out and about. Some close family, who hadn't breastfed themselves, considered breastfeeding to be something you did for a few weeks. The way they looked at me, or looked away with disapproval, hurt immensely. I wanted to be left alone to do what felt right for me. I was fortunate that my local friends were indifferent to my choices and let me be. They just accepted me for who I was. My mother-in-law made me feel particularly uncomfortable about it and often told me it was disgusting, they were too old and it wasn't good for their independence. They were five months old.

    Supermarket trips were a good way to get out of the house but people kept stopping me and cooing over the twins. I had a limited amount of time to get around the shop while they were still asleep or at least calm before their next feed or nappy change. I lived near a Waitrose that not only lacked baby changing facilities but had a toilet door that you couldn't get a twin pram through. I found it too stressful to venture to any further supermarkets and stay on top of their feeding and nappy changing. People who stopped me and even formed a queue at the pram, sent shivers down my spine. Lots of twin parents complain about all the attention they didn't want and the onslaught of questions. I was a very candid person but people often went too far.

"Are they natural?"

What sort of a question is delivered like that? How is a child unnatural? It's simply rude and inconsiderate. But this one, more than the others, I could at least understand and sometimes used the terminology myself. Not with strangers.

"Do twins run in your family?"

I liked to watch their expression as I replied with, "Is that a transparent attempt to ask me if I've battled with infertility?" I got this one from a funny you tube video called *mothers of multiples are freaks of nature, by mompetition.* It was hilarious and I only used this when the person interrogating me was rude.

"Did you have IVF?"

I once replied with, "What's your favourite position in bed with your husband?"

"Excuse me?" the woman gasped.

"Oh, I'm sorry; I thought we were asking very intimate questions—"

I don't include people who might be enquiring because they are considering going through IVF because I could tell who they were and was happy to help. I got annoyed with the nosey ones who just want to know whether there was something wrong with you. They even asked who had the problem. Another odd thing people can't seem to help saying is how easily they got pregnant.

"I get pregnant so easily but I've never had twins."

What do you say to that?

"Which one is your favourite?"

Is a recipe for serious twin-issues but people honestly believed you favour one over the other.

"The one not screaming at me," is my common response.

"Are they identical?" Is one of my favourites. How can a boy and a girl possibly be identical?

"No."

"Is it two girls?"

"No, the one in pink is a girl and the one in blue is a boy," I replied calmly, trying not to be patronising as I glanced at my watch.

"Oh, of course. So, are they identical?"

"I have two (or three) kids and I reckon that's harder than twins."

Why the competition? This was a truly annoying statement because it was completely different and I never have found an appropriate answer so an awkward silence always follows.

"I don't know how you manage," said while scanning my face for signs of not coping or imminent tears.

"I have to," or, "I'm a mother, we cope."

"You have a perfect family in one go - you're all done."

"Thant's very thoughtful for you to make that very important decision for me!"

This one only riles me because I want another child. It was interesting how people, even strangers in supermarkets, could feel free to make such life changing decisions for you. Twin mothers I knew who had a third or fourth are "tutted" at behind their backs. It was like pregnancy, whereby you became public property; strangers commented on you, voiced their opinion, touched your bump or children (and all I see is germs) and remark on them needing a hair cut or how your son looked like a girl - I would never say such things to anyone.

"So, you still decided to have another so soon?"

Unable to grasp the meaning of this at first, I soon came to realise that for most of the first year a lot of people thought I was pregnant again. Even if I had a full time mother's helper, exercised and dieted every single day, it would not aiter my stomach. As the physiotherapist and GP rightly informed me, I had an over-extended uterus, it was overstretched and would take eighteen months. I had to grin and bear the stomach and everyone pointing it out to me as if they were experts and I was merely a lazy slob. I isolated myself even further and did all my shopping on line, venturing out only when I was very desperate for company. Local playgroups were a godsend and I had made lots of lovely friends.

Chapter 7 – Adam and Kelly

Adam is by far the chattier one, while Kelly is more reserved and laid back, and it soon becomes apparent that they are very close and connected. The thing I shall always remember them for is their synchronised "pinkie picking" – they would both, during awkward or sad moments, feign distraction with the pinkie finger on their left hands and pick at the nail or skin. They always started this at precisely the same time, with the same pinkie finger and had no idea they were both mirroring each other. I could tell they were close.

Kelly had travelled to France with a boyfriend and was reluctant to return to England and face her family and friends with the news that they had separated. She was embarrassed to return home. Instead, she decided to work on the Channel Islands for a few weeks, recuperate and then face her family. She found work as a waitress for the summer but that didn't go quite to plan either when an evening in the rather cheesy Mermaid disco brought Adam into her life - she didn't go home for over two years. Adam was working a hundred hours a week in his uncle's hotel on the Island and they clicked instantly. They were twenty three years old.

Upon returning to England, work proved hard to secure. They lived with their parents for a while until they found work and somewhere to rent. Adam had to give a years notice on one job so they had to rent until they were able to move location. It didn't worry them; they had plenty of time to start a family and settle down – so they thought. They married in a local church when they were both twenty seven. Work still did not come easy and they both signed up to run a pub in Dorset. It went horribly wrong and they realised it was not for them within the first week of meeting a rather unpleasant owner who wouldn't give them their own front door key. They knew instantly that they could not have him in their daily lives – he wasn't supposed to be there. Miserably they shared too much wine on their first day there, knowing that it couldn't possibly work under the circumstances but this was their livelihoods tied up in one job. Bravely, they left within the first week with no money, no prospects and nowhere to live. They found work in hospitality for a large blue chip organisation and eventually managed to buy their own home. Now they felt settled and could have the family they wanted. They were thirty when Kelly fell pregnant. She had stopped taking the pill a couple of years earlier and was not actively trying so this came as an unexpected and pleasant surprise.

"It was a bank holiday, Good Friday, and I got this shitty pregnancy test out, not the posh one, the cheapest one, and looked for what looks like a line," she explains. "It was rubbish and hard to see. I asked Adam if he thought it looked like a line and he said no – so I chucked it in the bin. But something bothered me about it and I went back to have a second look, dug it out of the bin, and decided there was definitely a line. Well, nothing was open 'till ten, being a holiday, and I couldn't wait that long. I rushed out of the house and drove about until I found a Tesco's which was open earlier. They didn't have any pregnancy tests on the shelf so I had to wait for a pharmacist to come and help me, to my embarrassment, but it was a better test kit and it confirmed that I was pregnant. We were ecstatic."

Nine weeks later the bleeding began. The GP sent her for a check-up and scan, which she initially thought was a little over the top, but they proved right to be concerned about her and the baby. It was not developing. There was still a heart beat but it didn't look good. They brought her back a week later and the baby definitely hadn't developed and now there was no heartbeat. Kelly and Adam were given the option to have a D&C or miscarry naturally. They had been in and out of hospital almost three weeks already and since the pregnancy had happened easily for them they tried to be brave and told themselves that these things happen. It was a relief to just know where they stood.

"I decided it was better to just end the whole thing and try to move on rather than wait for more blood," Kelly tells me with heavy eyes. "I had the D&C on my thirtieth birthday."

There were a number of women having abortions on the same day and Kelly found this very difficult to deal with. Her coping mechanism was to get pregnant again before this babies due date, by Christmas, and she would be strong knowing that could happen - expecting no further problems. This was their misfortune, now everything would be all right, people didn't have repeated problems this young in life, did they? Christmas arrived without any pregnancy and Kelly was gutted. Another year passed – nothing. At this point they were trying very hard to get pregnant.

"I loathed that ovulation monitor," Adam seethes. "She used it constantly for two years, peeing on the stick every day, and it never seemed to work."

"My periods have always been sporadic," Kelly sighs. "But that stick—"

"She pissed on that stick constantly as we lived our lives around that taunting image of a smiley face – I hate that smiley face!" Adam says seriously but it still makes us laugh.

"Baby sex is shit," Kelly nods.

There seemed to be a flow of weddings in their social network and everyone was getting married then having children. They grew to dread these weddings and the news that was coming shortly thereafter. They all seemed to get pregnant easily and quickly. Kelly broke down at one wedding, unable to deal with her emotions any longer. It grew harder to talk to people and look them in the eye. It felt horrible. Kelly was in a really bad place by this time. Relationships with other people became strained and awkward and they closed in on themselves. They went in for tests and despite no obvious problems on either side, as is often the case, went ahead with IVF. They both chose to do the egg-share scheme and donated half of their eggs because they had decided not to freeze any embryos at this stage. There was no suspected problem with her eggs or his sperm so they didn't need to have ICSI either. It was a relief to them both to be starting IVF and actively doing something.

It didn't help that they both worked for the same boss who was snidy and inconsiderate in his comments to them and made them feel terrible. They had no choice but to confide in him, since they would both need so much time off in synchronisation. Not only did he comment on how easily he had impregnated his wife more than once but also told other people at work. His indiscretion and inconsideration ate away at them, more so for Adam, and it was a bitter pill to swallow.

Adam kept himself busy in the waiting room watching the other couples and trying to guess their situation and status. His eyes fell upon someone from work and they exchanged a silent look which seemed to say: "I know... You know... don't tell anyone but I can't acknowledge you." It was strange. Everyone was waiting for something and the atmosphere was horribly intense. Adam was intrigued with it and tried to guess, according to the level of nervousness, who was either just about to do or had done their wank. Trying to clock their status fascinated him and proved a good distraction. He noticed a side door for those who were not coping and they were discreetly escorted out.

"Kelly is squeamish so I had to jab her," Adam smiles. "She did do a couple herself but preferred me to do. I think the drugs helped her, she was a much happier and positive person while on them and they didn't seem to have much effect on her."

"I was just relieved and happy that something was happening. We had been trying for so long and nothing had happened but once we started IVF it all went very fast."

"We were peeved at having to wait an extra five weeks though because the couple we were donating to were on holiday!"

"Oh yes, that was annoying. It was the longest five weeks and I just kept thinking that I'm giving this woman my eggs, why should I have to wait?"

Adam grew concerned that they were trying to harvest more eggs than they normally would because she was on the egg-share scheme and she was more bloated than other women seemed to be. When it came to harvesting the eggs he was full of fear for Kelly's health. He struggled to focus on their rather good selection of porn and still do his part and then sat anxiously waiting for news of his wife.

"They butchered her, wanting to get as many eggs from her as possible and she looked really rough," Adam says angrily.

"Well, you can understand it, they don't want to let the other couple down and they said they'd had trouble retrieving the eggs. The follicles looked great on the scan but getting the eggs out was tough and I lost a lot of blood," Kelly nods.

They had twelve eggs and spilt them with the other couple. Six eggs each. It was a nervous wait until the following morning and Adam popped out briefly when they called with the news.

"I was feeling rather upbeat about it all," Kelly says. "But I didn't expect to hear what they told me – nothing had fertilised – nothing! One egg still stood a chance if they left it longer."

Kelly collapsed on the floor in a flood of tears. She desperately wanted to talk to someone but who do you share such a thing with? Eventually, she calmed down enough to speak on the phone with her mum and was able to get her head around it before Adam came home. All hopes were now pinned on this one remaining egg and what it decided to do. Later that day they received another call – it had fertilised. Kelly had little hope for this meagre egg that had taken much longer than normal to spark life. It was implanted but she held little expectation. They went on holiday with her parents to Scotland and on her birthday a pregnancy test showed that she wasn't pregnant. It was bearable, expected, and they had the immediate support of their family. They still hoped that the other couple who had shared their eggs had found success because they would have had ICSI as standard with donated eggs.

Their consultant did something strange then and put them on clomid, which is normally done before IVF, and if IVF failed, is unlikely to work. They couldn't understand this and eventually one of the nurses questioned it and they were told to stop. The nurse insinuated that IVF hadn't worked for the other couple either, knowing that they needed this information to be clear on what they needed to do. They needed another round of IVF with ICSI. It was hard having to face IVF again and they didn't have the money for it. It would be approximately £4700, plus £1000 for ICSI. Kelly's father offered to pay for the IVF but Adam couldn't bear that.

"I know it was well meaning but it felt totally wrong having the grandparents "buy" their grandchildren. But we did take a loan off him as long as he let us pay it all back," Adam sighed.

They purchased all the drugs for round two of IVF and then went in for tests, part way through, to check that Kelly had "down regulated."

"I decided to do a pregnancy test," Kelly sighs. "Just another shitty cheap one since it was unlikely anything had happened but I wanted to rule the possibility out. I had a line and was panic-stricken. I went and purchased a posh test to make certain – I was pregnant."

They had mixed emotions: excited to be pregnant without IVF but terrified of what the drugs might have done to the baby. The drugs were supposed to have stopped her ovulating so this was highly unlikely. She must have ovulated just before starting the drugs. They were told that the drugs were unlikely to affect the baby but their minds were not eased. They hadn't yet paid for anything above the drugs but the clinic still offered them a six week scan – they were very compassionate. The scan was disappointing and showed no heartbeat. They were crushed. All Kelly could see was another D&C and a wasted round of IVF but a week later there was a heartbeat and the baby seemed to be doing well. It would have been a very happy moment if it wasn't for the miserable attitude of the nurse.

"We got the dragon lady again," Adam laughs. "She was sour-faced and miserable. She told us not to get excited since most people lose the baby this early on. We could understand their need to be honest and realistic but she went overboard. She dashed our hopes completely and we felt negative."

"We asked her when we could feel as if we are out of the danger zone and she told us that would be when we were holding the baby. I understand that now but it was horrible to hear at the time," Kelly adds.

A further scan at eight weeks showed a perfectly healthy looking baby once more and they were told to go to their GP and schedule in the normal twelve week scan with the midwife. They were normal people now and could follow the normal route. Kelly had a lovely pregnancy until the end, when her high blood pressure caused concern for pre-eclampsia. Otherwise she was healthy. Her waters broke two weeks early, eleven on the night, and she was rushed in because of her blood pressure. When she arrived she was already nine centimetres dilated. They could see the baby's head and then it disappeared again. She had one arm up around the umbilical cold, which probably stopped the cord from strangling her, and was born with forceps – a perfectly healthy little girl named Gina. There were forty six babies that night and the ward was manic. Kelly needed to have her placenta surgically removed and was losing copious amounts of blood. There was no theatre free and the Polish doctor was determined to sort out the problem there and then: he stuck his large gloved hands up inside Kelly and began digging around. It was hurting Kelly and seemed a ridiculous thing to do at the time and Adam insisted that the doctor stopped and they managed to find a theatre for her, remove the placenta and give Kelly a blood transfusion. She didn't recover easily.

Kelly was on loads of drugs and combined with what she had been through her milk was slow coming through, taking four days, at which point Gina was starving. Breastfeeding was horrendous. They came home five days later, having had virtually no sleep on the ward, and gave Gina some formula they collected from a store open twenty four hours. Gina slept for twelve hours straight. They topped her up for the first three weeks, until Kelly's milk was flowing well, and then she could breastfeed solely for the next seven months. When Gina was nine months old Kelly had a slight bleed and assumed that her body was getting back into its normal cycle. She learned that she was pregnant again in April – the same date that she had gone through her first D&C. Another little girl, Josie, was born healthy and well nine months later. They constantly expected something to go wrong and still do even though both girls are growing well.

"Being a parent is flipping hard work," Kelly says stifling a yawn. "I love them so much but by goodness it's hard work! All that build up and stress just to get pregnant, fertilised, blah... blah...

blah... It's just constant worry and stress but it's such a joy and I would never change it. It's just so tiring!"

"We're really blessed," Adam smiles.

"I just feel bad for moaning about being tired or ill because of what I went through to have these, then I feel guilty for moaning about them even though other mum's moan," Kelly adds.

"But we're chuffed, delighted, privileged. We're never complacent now and certainly don't take things for granted."

"If I hadn't lost that first baby I don't think I'd appreciate these ones quite as much," Kelly says. "Looking back, it doesn't seem that long a time but when you're there it feels like forever. It really does make you appreciate them more. I never believed people when they talk about how easily they fell pregnant until Josie arrived. We narrowed it down to one time, didn't we, Adam?"

"Oh, definitely my birthday. I even joked whose it was because it just seemed so unlikely."

"If IVF hadn't worked it would have broken us for sure."

"No doubt – how do people get passed that? You go into yourself and turn on each other – it's very hard!"

Chapter 8 - The Magnanimous First Year

When it came to each stage of raising your children there seemed to be two main routes to take that were currently popular and, more often than not, clashed with what the older generation were told. For our parent's generation, weaning was three months, not the current six; potty training was anything from six months but certainly by eighteen months, instead of the current trend of two or three years. Many people adopted a route and then claimed it was the *only* way to do it. During a day at the park, we were discussing the eight month check with the health visitor who was returning to visit one baby because he had failed to clap during the check up. I didn't like the way a baby was treated like a performing monkey and dreaded my turn probably because I was concerned my twins were not as advanced as a singleton.

"I swear he has clapped before," said the mother with distress. "I feel awful. She's coming back!"

"So what? He's healthy, that's all that matters," I said, trying to calm her down.

"By the time they're eighteen, they'll all be clapping," another friend added and we all laughed.

I had made a circle of friends since the twins were born and enjoyed the socialising. I had missed out on NCT classes, which I later regretted, because we had done the TAMBA (Twins and multiple birth association) equivalent instead and decided not to pay for both. However, the twins club wasn't that friendly or welcoming and I failed to click with anyone there. I couldn't understand why and assumed it was because we were all so busy but even writing the newsletter didn't make me feel any closer to the group. I felt like an outsider. The friends the health visitor had put me in touch with were all close and connected by having had our babies at the same time. It was nice to spend time at each other's houses almost daily. Every time you got used to something and felt comfortable, it all changed and you moved on to yet another stage. Weaning was more complicated than I liked. Since breastfeeding was established, I felt no need to introduce solids early, and the world-wide recommendation, excessively pushed by health visitors, taking third world countries into account, was six months. Some of my friends would challenge the health visitor that six months was too long since we had clean water and sterilised equipment and lacked the third world unsanitary problems. There was no budging and we were made to feel that introducing solids before six months was child abuse. One of my friends in Wales was being told four months by her health visitor - it was silly. We had a lovely group of new mom's so we could reassure each other when we fell into the health visitors bad books. I had to remember that my twins were a month early so three months of age for them was only two gestational months. My mother-in-law was putting pressure on me.

"They cry so much because they are starving," she told me.

I had copious amounts of milk, they fed well, they were only three months old – or a gestational two months - there was no rush. She was relentless and even enlisted my sister-in-law to comment on how hungry they seemed, a word-for-word repeat of what I had been told the previous day. It was blatantly obvious they had been discussing me and, like most people, I detest that. From the start I had been concerned that I couldn't feed my babies properly, in one way or another. After two weeks of pressure I gave in and introduced baby rice. I was uncertain, lacking in confidence and my mother-in-law was adamant that they needed it – I was starving them. She has this whole thing about babies being hungry and needing more, as had been her experience as a mother (she switched to formula with her babies very early on in order to measure quantities and I completely understood such pressure). I knew this was not personal towards me, she had put similar pressure on her friend's daughter who, sadly, trusted her advice too much and stopped breastfeeding early on and switched to formula in order to measure it!

My midwife told me that many women were unable to trust that their bodies could do what nature required and meet the needs of their baby and it reassured me immensely. I felt sad that my mother-in-law didn't have a midwife like mine at the time. A good midwife made all the difference – as did a bad one. It was rare that it truly didn't work. My mother-in-law helped me feed them solids and loved it. I suddenly realised that the pressure was perhaps more because she wanted to be involved in feeding her grandchildren. However, I knew their little stomachs were struggling, even though they ate it, and they were in pain. After a week I couldn't bear it any longer and stood my ground, was true to my own instincts, and gave up solids.

Our relationship turned even sourer. She didn't understand why I had a problem and nothing I said made sense to her. I wish I had been strong enough to tell her to mind her own business - I was a shadow of my former self – and a people pleaser. Motherhood overwhelmed me, left me insecure, uncertain and petrified of everything. I never knew if I was doing the right thing, information was conflicting, and I was obviously useless. I felt only pressure and received no positive help from James or his family. I had been outcast from my own family for years for marrying a snob (four out of five children had been cut off for petty reasons – it was how my father worked). I tried again to get in touch with my parents but they were not interested, just as they hadn't been with their other grandchildren. I harboured huge resentment that my mother had refused every attempt to meet up during and after pregnancy and I desperately needed and wanted her. We had not fallen out over anything bad and there was no reason for it and I hated the fact that she refused to see me when I clearly needed her so much. It was cruel and unnecessary and it made me dislike my mother-in-law even more too for not covering the space my own mother had left.

My health visitor was furious with me for introducing solids so early but she was nothing compared to the wrath of my mother-in-law who constantly told me how I was tolerated and wasn't good enough for her son. I used to laugh at how I could be called a snob and common at the same time but it wasn't so funny anymore. I desperately needed a mother figure and she was all I had. She came for two days a week and stayed overnight at my sister-in-laws, which upset me because it was clear she didn't want to stay here and complained about the messy house. I knew that she was only tolerating me for the day so she could be near her grandchildren and had no intention of spending time with just me and her son. It hurt that she would socialise with my sister-in-law and no doubt spend the evening discussing all the bad choices I had made that day. I wanted desperately to be liked by her, as she liked my sister-in-law, but I could never seem to get that. I thought of 'Meet The Fockers' again.

This made me hate and resent my own mother more for not being there for me. My family was dysfunctional and should be on Eastenders with all the drama. There was so much bitterness that no one could talk to each other and we simply brought out the worst in each other. My father had five children and put myself and my youngest sister into private school to do better and "escape the slums of Birmingham." I went onto college and university, my youngest sister dropped out, and I was the only sibling to do well in my career. Then I was cut off for being a snob and I do not think I am mean spirited or snobby in anyway – I just wanted to do well. I felt betrayed for doing exactly what my father wanted.

I tried to make the most of having my mother-in-law here but at a time when I felt most vulnerable I was with a woman who resented and disliked me – her feelings were too strong to hide and it was obvious. I felt as if she was watching my every move for fault and criticism. I didn't like the things she said about her friends when she opened up to me and it made me wonder what on earth she said about me. I ignored the looks of disgust at the dog hair everywhere and the cat food spilled on the floor. I was a complete slob in her eyes. I was hygienic but messy and with twin babies, a dog and cat, my house could never be as clean as hers. She called me a slag once and when I looked at her, eyes saucer-wide, she explained that it is what she and her friends called women who didn't care how they looked and dressed in their pyjamas all the time. Although I was breastfeeding around the house in my pyjamas a lot I also went out to playgroups almost daily and I did wear clothes for such events. I swallowed many hurtful comments.

I hated dummies/pacifiers and reluctantly introduced them because of their colic. I was determined not to use them for long, especially because of the dog and cat hair, and didn't want the battle so many people seemed to have getting dummies off four year olds. I made them go cold turkey when they were about five months old and my mother-in-law couldn't cope with it. We both ended up in tears with the stress and almost having a massive fall out. She would not stay downstairs while I tried to sooth the babies and kept running in, all ruffled, angry and tearful because of what I was doing "to the poor things." I had no choice but to give the babies their dummies back – she was hysterical and making it worse. For once I knew what I was doing and waited until she had gone.

    I knew what to do, had talked about it enough with the local mums and knew what would work with my babies. I cut their dummies, told then they were broken and let them hold them. They sucked, got nothing out of it, and understood. They again cried for thirty minutes before bed but I soothed one while James soothed the other – what I had expected his mother to do. At least James always did what I asked, without question, because he trusted my opinion as far as our children were concerned. My son never moaned again. My daughter struggled more and had trouble getting off to sleep if she woke up in the night. I let her sleep with me for two nights and taught her how to sooth herself back to sleep. After two nights it was all accomplished. No dummies. All it took was a bit of resolve to get through that first half hour. I was a big believer that children, even that young, can see it in your eyes if you were going to fold. If I did something, I stuck to it, and cutting up all the dummies was the best way to ensure I didn't give in. Something must have told me not to cut them up with the mother-in-law helping.

    I wasn't the only one struggling with the birth of the twins: everything electrical collapsed within the first few months. The tumble dryer was first to go, then the washing machine, fridge, freezer, kettle, vacuum, dehumidifier – it would have been comical if the vast expense hadn't wiped the smiles from our faces. It was always something that was essential. The dehumidifier kept the mould off the windows, the dryer was essential now my laundry had increased, it saved on ironing and took less time than hanging items up to dry, especially with washable nappies that failed to do what I was sold – they took three days to dry, not one, so had to be tumble dried to finish them off – completely against the environmentally friendly approach I was striving to achieve. I gave up on washable nappies during the day after about five months, when outfits wouldn't fit over their bottoms unless I purchased the next size up. Disposable nappies with twins were far easier and I soon got over my environmental concerns – I wasn't supermom. I continued to use washable nappies overnight for a few more months. As time passed, my confidence returned and I began to have a clearer picture of what I wanted to be and how I wanted to do things. It became clear to me that my lack of confidence and low self-esteem had turned me into an over-sensitive, touchy grouch. I started weaning again at four and a half months – a gestational three and a half months – because the pressure hadn't ceased from the mother-in-law and this was a compromise.

Throughout the first year they would have slept through the night if colic, teething and winter bugs hadn't bothered them. They were good sleepers but these things had conspired to keep us alert and awake the entire year. I continued to go to bed at the same time as the twins and James watched them until midnight - they never settled. It was the only way I could get any sleep but that left no time to go out, make phone calls or have any adult interaction. James and I only spoke to discuss chores that needed doing. I finally called the TAMBA helpline (the twins and multiple births association) before I went insane and they gave me some great tips on how to get more sleep since they kept waking each other up. In order to break these bad habits we kept a table on the wall detailing when they awoke, why and how long it took to settle them because we were too tired to remember anything. It worked, we figure out who was doing what, ignored the attention seeking parts and took control.

By five months Chris was crawling and darted about the floor like a little ferret. I was lucky because I only had to keep him out of mischief since Beth was perfectly content watching him. By the time Chris could pull himself up and was trying to master walking, Beth was crawling, so I could focus on her. When Chris had mastered walking at nine months Beth was starting to master pulling herself up and moving around the sofa and tables: once more only one to chase. Chris was a little dare-devil, into everything, and drove me crazy but Beth liked watching him and it made my life easier. It was a different story later on when they could both walk and darted off in opposite directions. One would head towards the river and one towards the road. I swallowed my heart often and was far from a relaxed and contented mother. It was a relief to see other mothers equally as stressed as they chased one or two toddlers at alarming speed.

    I didn't enjoy my first Christmas with five month old twins. I was literally left holding the babies, on the sofa, for three days and nights. I was bored stiff, suffocating and desperate for some fresh air. No one would have the twins off me, not even for a couple of hours. I was getting fed up with my lack of space to the point I almost resented the twins. We were again at my parents-in-law and I did not feel comfortable. We were routine maniacs – it was the only way to survive with twins. I never used to be a fan of routine, preferring flexibility, until they actually arrived. You had to be strict and disciplined or chaos ensued. This meant meal times and attempted nap times had to occur as scheduled, without fail. It was a coping mechanism and we were coping by using it.

    My brother and sister-in-law were not successful with their IVF and there was an understandable atmosphere everyone was trying to ignore. This possibly added to my mother-in-laws resentment towards me for being the daughter-in-law with the children. Life is ironic because her life would have been so different if my sister-in-law had been the one who provided her with grandchildren. It would have been the perfect family situation for them and James and I would have just been pushed out. James did not have a good relationship with his parents but his brother was very close to them. It was ironic.

    Trying to decide when to eat was difficult. No one wanted to eat before six on the evening but James and I explained the twins will not be well behaved that late and his parents wanted them with us at Christmas dinner. They were normally asleep by six thirty and expecting them to last a further two hours was unrealistic. Everyone was over-precious about asking us when they could do things, obviously resenting the timings being dictated by us, and it was unpleasant. No one seemed to understand that it wasn't us dictating the day it was the plain fact that we had two babies and they needed to sleep and feed regularly. There was another twin mum I knew who had the same problem with this lack of understanding at Christmas and her sister-in-law verbally attacked her and they had a full on screaming match.

It was bizarre because accommodating different ages at events such as Christmas; be it babies, toddlers, the elderly, is not about dictatorship but individual requirements. My parents were always really good with that and never made an issue of anything. Conversations in our family were more along these lines: "well, we can't eat then because the toddlers will be too tired and won't behave, and Uncle John will be too pissed, we need him to pass out after the meal not before." No one was ever made to feel as if they were dictating, it was all about accommodation. I missed my family even more, despite how loud and chaotic the day was with eighteen of us crammed into my mother's house, but it was always nice as long as you left before the drunken nastiness set in on everyone.

If this wasn't enough to contend with I had to face the sixty-year-old cousin of my mother-in-law who cornered me alone in the kitchen.

"You need to do something about your weight," she declared, arms folded.

"I have five month old twins and the physiotherapist said it won't come off yet no matter what I do. I can't diet while I'm breastfeeding," I replied resenting feeling the need to explain my weight.

"But you must think of your health for the sake of the children, even if your weight doesn't bother you. They need you around."

I looked at her in disbelief. I was only 9lbs heavier than pre-pregnancy but it was all belly and boobs. "Thanks for telling me but I'm fine with my body," I insisted stony-faced.

"Well, your husband still has to want you!"

At which point I walked out the room and told James, his brother and wife about the conversation. They seemed awkward and I suspected they had all been in on it and had agreed she would be the best person to pass this much needed advice onto me. I could just imagine everyone talking about me and how big I had become. I felt sick. James often told me that he "didn't do fat." I wanted to scream, "have the children then, so I can do some exercise!" I found this woman deeply unpleasant, as does her estranged daughter and several ex-husbands, and once she accidentally reversed into my mother-in-law's car and rather than lose her no claims bonus, planed to force another driver to go into the back of her by slamming on her breaks, making them responsible for the cost of the damage.

"You aren't serious?" I asked, shocked that she would even think such a thing.

"Yes, I bloody am, I'm not paying for it!" She retorted as if that made perfect sense.

"But you did it, you have to take responsibility. What about that other car? They might have a dog in the boot or children in the back!"

She leaned forwards, like a witch, to add conviction to her next words, "Well, Grace, that's just life!"

I found her so evil she made me shiver and I never found out if she actually went ahead with this. I felt as if I was surrounded by inconsiderate, selfish and nasty people and it was getting to me. I didn't even have a loving relationship with James.

During the Christmas meal I grew increasingly uncomfortable and was told how this witch-woman (the cousin) had a dream that I gave her my son and asked her to raise him for me. I silently listened to the details of her dream, seething, as everyone watched for my reaction which I deliberately kept nonchalant. It turned out, according to an account by my mother-in-law given a week later, that it wasn't really a dream but a conversation they had shared. I couldn't believe she thought it was acceptable to share this with me and made me wonder how bad the parts she missed out were. They had been discussing my inability to raise my children – particularly my son – who I apparently failed to understand. They had discussed me asking them to raise him because I couldn't cope with two. I hated the way they talked about me and preferred it to be behind my back. I did not want to hear such conversations repeated to me.

The twins were both lactose intolerant, like their father had been as a baby, and couldn't stomach cow dairy. I gave them goat dairy, it was easier to digest the lactose, was readily available and I saw no point in letting their little stomachs suffer – cow dairy made them snotty and gave them terrible diarrhoea. I read plenty of negative things about cow dairy and had always preferred goat. I soon tired of expressing my milk for their cereal and my confidence continued to return. I was becoming more comfortable with motherhood by six months, despite the mother-in-law.

"Whatever you say Grace," she would say resentfully. "If that's how *you* want to do it."

She did this in front of other people, deliberately making me look bad and to prove a point she had obviously been discussing with them behind my back. I hated being made out to be something I was not. There was so much to do and every time she got into the swing of it she vanished to France for weeks and everything was different upon her return. I showed her what I did and understood she felt as if I were being bossy. I understood her but she had no idea about the type of person I was.

My breastfeeding days came to an end rapidly and much sooner than I liked.

We stayed with the parents-in-law in France and it was incredibly stressful. They made me feel awkward about wanting to eat at my usual times: noon and five. They ate much later, often finishing at ten and I couldn't do that every day. I was far too tired and often in bed by nine and I needed food earlier to produce sufficient milk. They accused me of dictating and being difficult and couldn't, or didn't want to understand.

I could understand this since they had hired a nanny for each son from birth until they were sent away to boarding school at five and therefore she wasn't a hands on mother like me, had forgotten everything or advice had since changed. We were polar opposites. The most traumatic part of the holiday was when my mother-in-law had this bright idea that a local physiotherapist could treat the twins and help with their lactose intolerance – removing a lot of the congestion on their chests – scaring me with stories of future lung problems. I was happy to try anything to ease the comfort of the twins, and cranial osteopathy had previously worked wonders for their colic, but I was not expecting what he did.

It was the cruellest and most gruesome thing I had ever witnessed: he pinned the babies down, one at a time, and attempted to spend ten minutes banging and compressing their chests, choking them and forcing them to cough up spit and gunk. They were terrified and distraught by it and so was I. He was angry with me for yelling at him to stop and snatching my babies away. My mother-in-law hadn't stayed in the room, saying she couldn't watch it, but I was glad I was there to put an end to it. It was doing no good at all but hurting them. What upset me the most was that he said one treatment was useless; it needed a course, which was of no use to me since I was only in France for a fortnight. I couldn't have it done in the UK because, and this really made my heart sink, it was illegal. He was saying all this and I hadn't spoken a word because I had ended it prematurely and had absolutely no intention of continuing with such a barbaric treatment. The twins were still shaking and crying hysterically. I refused to let my mother-in-law hold them; I held them both tight to my chest and felt consumed with guilt as I held back the tears.

There were many other little things, as there often is, such as the time I asked her not to spray insect killer in the house while the twins were there. It was hot and the flies were everywhere but James and I were having fun zapping them with the electronic tennis rackets and got rid of them manually. The twins were so little and those sprays contain terrible ingredients often banned in the UK but not in France. I was not the sort of person who used aerosols or sprays in the home – all natural and ecover for me. His parents were not happy that we had asked this, that was clear, but I still expected them to respect our point and consider the babies lungs. The following morning my mother-in-law made a dramatic point of carrying the insect spray from the fireplace mantelpiece and returning it to the cupboard, so only I could see while I was breastfeeding, making it clear she had sprayed it that very morning. I said nothing – what was the point? I knew it was deliberately to spite me – I saw the way she looked at me with glee in her eyes - why make such an effort to ensure I saw her carry it past me otherwise? It seemed like such a cruel thing to do. I felt so sick and took my babies into the garden as soon as I could for some fresh air. I couldn't believe anyone would do such a thing.

All this stress and the food too late in the day caused my milk supply to dwindle. I hated them for their lack of support, especially James, who had promised not to let them bully me on the holiday he forced me to go on when I begged him to say we couldn't go. He understood what was happening, saw me crying when I tried to feed them but had no milk, would tell me how sorry he was that they were being like this but his sympathy meant nothing to me when I couldn't feed my children and he wouldn't stand up for me. I stayed quiet because I couldn't handle the confrontation that would follow. I had given them cups of water to drink from six month of age and they soon insisted on cups instead of breast. I wished I had the courage to just stand up for myself and do what I wanted but I knew James would get angry with me for causing trouble. I couldn't help but wonder if it had been her mission to put an end to her grandchildren being breastfed at ten months of age and save them from a life of dependence. I started drinking instead.

His mother kicked us out for two days in the blazing heat, in order to clean the house and shut it up for their return to England. I was furious but still couldn't bring myself to talk to his parents while I was a guest in their house. It was hard to keep the twins out of the sun, as we spent two long days on a beach, and I was worried sick they would get sun stroke. I told James he had to stand up to his mum and say we couldn't be kicked out of the house during a heat wave with ten month old babies. He lost it – with me. I realised that he would rather have a row with me than his mother. He just wanted me to stop moaning and accept everything regardless of how it made me of the twins feel.

I told him I wanted a divorce and it was the most unpleasant argument we had ever had. That I had ever had! We hissed at each other on the beach so that other people couldn't hear us. All I could see was the well-being of my children and he didn't seem to care about that. We eventually made up, for the sake of the children, and apologised to each other. I had lost respect for him and despised his weakness, as I saw it, to do the right thing for his children. In over two weeks James and his parents refused to look after the twins so I could do a walk with Fudge, cycle with James or simply sleep. James had freedom and space, I did not and I resented it.

I felt unsupported and misunderstood – what was vitally important to me meant nothing to anyone else in the family. Why couldn't they just let me be a good mother to my children and respect that? I certainly wasn't doing a bad job. By the end of the holiday Beth was refusing to breastfeed due to the lack of milk. Within a month of that holiday my breastfeeding days were over. I had no milk left and the children wanted cups of more readily available milk. It broke my heart. I wasn't ready to stop. I began to descend into darkness.

I'd never been a baby person and always preferred toddlers. People told me it would be different with my own but it was not: they were largely boring and the work was mundane. Give me a toddler and here I come! I loved it from about eight months when they were turning into little people and developing a character. I was coming into my element. I was much happier as a mother and no one could make me feel stupid or incompetent anymore. Strong opinions against my choice no longer bothered me because I was confident with my knowledge and decision. I had been a nanny and auntie to toddlers and was in my comfort zone. I realised how my insecurity had given strength to other people's opinions and how irrelevant and trivial they would have been if I had merely had more confidence in myself. It was an eye-opener. I had become petty and silly. It was time to change.

As sleep became more available I started to become a nicer person but James was still nasty and the way he spoke to me became increasingly vile. I knew he was struggling with parenthood as much as I was and I didn't make a big deal about his outbursts or treatment towards me. He often turned on me when stressed or unhappy – I was used to it. I swallowed the insults, held them deep down, and let them eat away at my self-esteem. No arguments occurred and I took to going to bed with the twins since I was so exhausted and it helped avoid the insults. We barely saw each other.

Since all I seem to say is "Fudge, heel," or "Fudge, come," or, "Fudge, nooooo!" It was no surprise that Fudge was the first word both twins uttered as opposed to mummy or daddy. It was impossible to keep track of what day of the week it was, let alone what had happened that morning or the day before so I kept a diary of all their little moments. James was hoping to get a promotion as a partner in his law firm and had become increasingly stressed when his review was delayed. He told me this was why he was being horrible and why he had me in tears most evenings – our holiday in France had taken its toll on our relationship and we hadn't recovered. I was drinking far too much wine now I was no longer breastfeeding.

If I was in a good mood, had a lovely day with the children, he wouldn't stop until I was in tears. He chipped away at me until I broke no matter how determined I was to remain happy. Each day, I set my mind to going to bed smiling, no matter how he was when he got home from work, but I never manage it and my depression deepened. I was happy during the day, with the twins and friends, but the whole atmosphere changed when he got home. I hated the way things were and just wanted to enjoy my time with the children. I knew things were bad between us and there seemed to be nothing I could do about it. I was losing my respect for him and becoming increasingly resentful that he was ruining what should be a precious time for me. When he wasn't nasty, he was introvert and withdrawn – I couldn't pull him back – and knew he was also depressed. Each morning he apologised, each evening he started on me again. He promised me that it was just work and he would be all right soon enough. I clung to that promise.

He didn't get the promotion and his behaviour became intolerable. I couldn't talk to him. Sometimes I would stand up for myself, in a calm and rational manner, which seemed to make him angrier and made him crave conflict. He always said sorry and always did it again. It was torture. I begged him to do counselling, alone or together, he wouldn't hear of it. Convinced he was suffering from depression, I begged him to go to the doctors. He refused. The hateful way he looked at me broke my heart and the way he spoke to me sent my blood cold. I called his only two friends, who he barely saw, and begged them to talk to him, explaining that he was depressed about his review. I didn't know what else to do. They called a couple of times, he wouldn't answer, and they gave up. I knew I had lost him and had no idea how to get him back.

    His parents were due back from another spell in France and his mother wanted to spend the usual two days a week with her grandchildren. I didn't want to stop her seeing them and loathed the thought of being a controlling mother but wanted to keep myself safe from further hurtful comments. It was always full on and I dreaded spending so such time with her, especially under the circumstances. If she had been able to watch the twins while I had a bath or slept then at least I wouldn't be with her constantly but she couldn't, or wouldn't, do this. I asked my reverend, upon Jude's advice, to come round and help despite the fact I had barely ever been to church but we needed an outsider and he was a lovely man. I explained what I needed and with his guidance got James to communicate and work with me about finding a solution. It was the only way I could force James to discuss it with me.

    I felt bullied by his mother but did acknowledge that I didn't know how much of this was paranoia or my over-sensitive emotions. One thing that was clear was how different she was in front of other people. I hated afternoons, the twins were cranky and I was exhausted by the end of the day. Plus, I treasured the peaceful afternoon nap they were finally taking together. We told her she could visit in the mornings and join me at the local play groups, ensuring I was never alone with her in the house. Or, she could see them any evening or weekend when James was around. She refused to visit then, to my relief, and I knew then that I may be oversensitive but I wasn't imagining her treatment towards me – it was about being alone with me more than seeing the grandchildren or she would have come to the playgroups like other grandparents. I felt like a toy she enjoyed playing with.

I needed to be strong for the children and couldn't do that with both her and James putting me down. Lots of other grandparents went to the groups but she did it once or twice then never came in the week again. She found the occasional Saturday that she could fit us in, she was obviously upset, and this made me even more convinced that there was something unhealthy going on. I began to wonder if it wasn't bullying but more about control and she was trying to look like a doting grandmother to her friends. A friend told me that many women embraced becoming a grandmother while others saw it as a demotion in status and I wasn't helping matters by having an opposite approach to mothering.

She often called me a hippy, not in a nice way, and often the word disgusting appeared in the same sentence. I could see that I gave her no power and never sought her advice – I had spent a lifetime not having parents and was independent. At least now I could focus on James. His temper was fowl and the way he treated me and even the twins was worrying. He was a bully, coming down especially hard on Chris, prompting me to stand up to him – protecting them. One evening I screamed at him to release Chris, who was refusing to lie still for a nappy change, and James was hurting him and swearing at him as he pinned him down by the throat. Chris was terrified - so was I. This was the turning point for me when I no longer stayed passive, swallowing all the abuse, and began fighting back. James had suffered with depression from the age of ten and, despite admitting to that, continued to refuse to address it. I turned to wine or writing in order to escape him and continued with the early nights. I avoided confrontation unless he was hurting the kids and tried to find enough energy to look after the children alone and reduce how much he did since he wasn't coping. He was losing control. I focused on the children during the day, went to bed soon after them, and tried to be a good mother. I cherished them.

After their first birthday, I put my foot down with James and insisted that he had to take them out for a few hours at the weekend and give me some space – I was exhausted. Also, I had now gained weight as a result of all the wine and comfort eating. I was desperate to hit the gym and get rid of it – he had to give me time at the weekend to do that as I didn't have the energy to go in the evenings after chasing the twins all day. I also needed to clear my head to try and sort our marriage out and only space would give me the means to do so. I felt everything was on me and I was incapable of coping. I started to see myself as a bad mother, as I was frequently told by James because of my drinking, and considered how much better off my children would be without me. The guilt was terrible. These thoughts were strong, scared me and I grudgingly went on anti-depressants.

My hormones were a mess and since my happy breastfeeding hormones had left I had descended into a dark and scary depression that toyed with my mentality. Combined with the way James was treating me I grew increasingly convinced that I was a terrible mother and person. It made me drink more and hate myself more because of it. I never drank to the point of being unable to look after the children, and only two or three times a week, certainly not daily but his abuse and the guilt made it so much worse. Extreme emotions raged through me and gripped me one by one; terror, grief, loneliness, guilt, anger, bitterness. By the end of the evening I was insane because tiredness made it worse. I sobbed to Jude on the phone, telling her I was mentally damaged, that I could feel it, and didn't know what to do. It was a scary place to be and each week it got worse.

My body was not functioning properly: sugar levels were scarily low and I often had severe diarrhoea. My bowels went under the slightest stress, which was daily with James. Often it was so sudden I failed to make it upstairs to the toilet. This both scared and shamed me. James looked at me with disgust and I shrivelled up inside. I sometimes passed blood and went to the GP thinking it was bowel cancer but she said it was just the damage from pre-eclampsia and hopefully my body would sort itself out soon enough. Part of me was still scared of dying on the twins and leaving them with a selfish introvert father.

I was a fairly positive person, when I wa healthy, and had always handled James's depression well. However, throw twin babies at me all day long and I had nothing left to give him. I was starting to realise just how much time and attention he needed and

I couldn't provide it. He constantly complained that he got no attention. I was beginning to think straight at last, the anti-depressants were helping, and I knew that I needed a break. I wanted him to love me, to feel loved, not hated. I was hit hard with the realisation that not one person around me, since the birth of my twins, loved me. Not James, not his family, and my new friends were still new but seeing them kept me going as I tried to pretend everything was good. Everyone else lived too far away. All I had ever wanted was children and now that I had them everything was going horribly wrong.

He took them out on a Saturday for a couple of hours two or three times (since they had turned one) to daddy's group and he obviously didn't want to do it. He plodded along grudgingly with whatever plans I made but without any joy or enthusiasm. It broke my heart - this was not how it should be. It was awful being with someone who seemed to hate me and knowing he was my husband. I tried not to focus on it. I lost over a stone and loved being back at the gym. When I arranged a babysitter and booked a weekly meal together, he would cause an argument, no matter how hard I tried to make it a nice evening. I felt persecuted and trapped with nowhere to go and no one to turn to. I tried to accept this as part of the depression and keep it in perspective but it was incredibly hard to do so.

"You are such a kill joy!" I moaned one morning after avoiding his wrath the evening before. "You hate seeing me happy, don't you?"

Always apologetic in the mornings, he hung his head in shame. "I know. It's horrible to admit and I wish I felt differently but you're right: I don't like you being happy because I can't be. It won't happen again. I'm sorry."

It always happened again. I tried to be sympathetic now I had a firmer understanding of depression but it was hard work. Once a week I organised a night out just for us because I was part of a token ring babysitting system, where we babysat for each other in return for tokens. I had earned double tokens for all the weekends I had done so had plenty to use up. It was a wonderful system. James sabotaged every date and had no intention of having a nice evening. My first mother's day came and went without any effort despite his mother reminding him and telling him to make it special for me. My resentment towards him grew and I stopped organising our failed nights out.

Chapter 9 – Mark and Susan

Susan is a petite woman, pretty and serene, with strong Christian values. Her conviction and integrity is admirable. She adores her husband Mark, who she met at the Christian Union at university during fresher's week. They dated and knew straight away they were meant for each other. My first impression of Mark is a good looking quiet, polite gentleman who makes a good cup of tea. However, I found him surprisingly talkative and open and immediately saw his love and dedication to Susan. They are both obviously very respectful and supportive of each other. They are a lovely couple. Mark was a year ahead at university and when he graduated he made sure he found a job nearby and they continued to date. From the start they planned marriage and children – it was all so clear and simple.

They were due to go on holiday to the Lake District after Susan's graduation and they purchased an engagement ring together: which Mark then snatched away from her and placed in his pocket with a knowing smile. The next day they went on holiday and Susan was a bag of nerves knowing what was coming and wondering when he was going to give her the ring. They had gone with five other couples and alone time was limited. One day, Mark announced that he and Susan were off for a walk and they left before anyone could encroach on their time. As they walked along the sandy beach Susan wondered if this was the moment and she realised what a lovely day and place it was – this would be perfect. But, they were not yet alone. Some of their friends had also decided to take a walk, suspecting nothing of what was going on, and spotted them strolling along the sand. They called out and Mark lowered his head and pulled Susan along in the hope of shaking them off.

Finally alone, Mark went down on one knee in the wet sand and proposed. It was a wonderful moment and, of course, Susan accepted. A year later they married. It was to be a beautiful church wedding and reception but five weeks before the big day Susan lost her father and it was a massive blow. It was too late to cancel or reschedule the wedding and Susan was in no mood to have a big ordeal now – she wanted plain and simple – but she had to go along with it. It was the hardest day of her life being both the saddest and the happiest. Her father had been sick from an early age and his mother was told that he wouldn't make it to fifty. A fighter and loving man, he partied hard on his fiftieth Birthday with nothing but joy. Five years later he had an unexpected heart attack and just missed walking his beloved daughter down the aisle. Susan was broken-hearted but this was not to be the biggest challenge for her and Mark to face in their new life together.

Three years later they were told that they could not have children naturally. One thing Susan knew for certain was that she did not want IVF: she battled with creating life in such a way and the thought of disregarding living embryos was too much to bear. She would not - could not - do IVF. The doctors insisted that it would be their only option. Since they were only twenty seven they did not qualify for NHS funding so it would cost them money they could not easily acquire. It didn't help that their consultant was flippant and inconsiderate to the point of being obnoxious; rather unhelpfully informing them that a bulldog has millions of sperm! They couldn't bear to be treated by such a man who made them feel like just another number and problem to be solved - it left a bad taste. He wanted to get them listed and ready to go there and then: money was to be made. They declined.

They considered adoption and went to PACT (Parents And Children Together) to learn more about adopting children from vulnerable backgrounds. After visiting several clinics and attending some talks on adoption, there was no doubt in Susan's mind that this was right for her – it felt obvious and she could really make a difference. They were in a room full of people and wondered why they were all there; perhaps they had fertility problems too; perhaps they wanted to help a child who had no home; perhaps they were too old to have their own children. Their minds raced with wonder. These people held secrets that would remain their own and it became clear that adoption was all about the children being adopted, not about any personal need to have children. But Mark wasn't as keen as Susan and needed to think about it.

Mark was training for the London marathon and running miles while shouting angrily at God for the unfairness of their infertility. Running enabled him to deal with his anger and think things through. There had been a time, when they were on holiday in Edinburgh, when Susan's period was two weeks late. Instead of enjoying Edinburgh, they walked aimlessly around, unable to think of anything except if this was it: had their time to become parents finally arrived? He finds this very difficult to talk about because they were soon to be very disappointed.

"When you really want children," Mark tells me, "it dominates your mind and every thought that exists."

Mark struggled with his emotions since he was the one unable to give his wife the natural conception she craved and his fertility problems left a gaping hole within his heart as the anger raged within. It was also difficult for him to talk to Susan because he knew how determined she was not to have IVF but he desperately wanted his own biological child and this made him feel guilty. He felt that not only was he to blame but he was being selfish by not wanting to adopt. He was also gutted that they had decided to wait so long before trying for children, not imagining it might be a problem, choosing instead to spend time enjoying each other's company first. This weighed heavily upon his mind when they found conception beyond their reach.

Those little faces he saw looking out to him at PACT tugged at his heart and the guilt rose to immeasurable levels. Eventually, he was able to raise the subject with Susan and his emotions overcame him – he broke down in tears, which was something he had never done before. However, this enabled Susan to realise just how much it meant to him – but now their goals and desires were very different. They agreed to compromise: one round of IVF then adoption. They investigated alternative clinics until they found the right one. They immediately warmed to a consultant who had published over a hundred scientific papers and was passionate about prevention of infertility and making assisted conception treatments more physiological, safer and affordable.

It was this almost holistic approach and care towards a woman's body that Mark respected. He could tell that they cared about his wife and what her body was about to go through and appreciated that respect and understanding. They had a minimal approach to the drugs and ensured that the best possible health options were considered instead of just thrusting full-on IVF drugs at them. Their obstetrician was also highly impressive: a pioneer in ultrasound diagnosis in medicine and many of his 3D and 4D ultrasound images had been used in TV documentaries. Mark admired his academic achievements and to have such a man consulting with them was an honour – they were undoubtedly superb people and they both knew instantly that this was the place for them.

They spoke with friends with various experiences of infertility, adoption and IVF. They talked, cried, denied the problem, ignored the issue and prayed... prayed... prayed. Having made the decision and chosen the clinic, they now had to raise £4,500. Mark's parents offered to pay for the treatment but he refused their help. This was his problem and his issue to deal with; he had to take responsibility and charge of his own life. He also didn't want them to be disappointed at losing their money for nothing if it didn't work. He had to raise it himself – and he worked hard to do so. On ethical grounds they chose only to fertilise two embryos despite repeated warnings that this lowered their chances of success. However, the clinic supported them every step of the way and worked hard to ensure optimum results.

Initially, Susan was insistent that she would need counselling because of her attitude towards IVF and she couldn't bear to know, or face handling the emotional aspect of knowing about every single, painful, scientific step. As it turned out she was eventually able to face it with her own faith and strength, seven years after they were married, five years after they knew they had no choice. It took them both years to accept it as a path. While building up to IVF she encountered a great deal of emotions and struggled with some people's comments. For example, she needed new windows in the front of the house and some friends told her not to waste her money but put it aside for IVF instead. She was angry. Why should she? Why couldn't she have new windows AND a child? Lots of people get jobs done around the house before they start a family why should she have to be different?

They hadn't had to choose so why should she? It was not fair that she should have to face this and make such financial decisions when other people didn't have to.

It upset Mark when Susan's first injection went wrong - the advice she had been given was inaccurate and she had a bad response to it. He watched her put on a brave face and deal with it "like the trooper she is." A friendly doctor helped her with the second injection, which was better, but they were not easy to do and caused immense pain and problems for her. It broke Mark's heart and yet again he wished she didn't have to do this: he was making her go through it all while he sat and watched. The guilt continued to rush over him. It was all very difficult and he will never forget the symptoms she went through and how brave he thought she was. He loved and admired her more than ever.

In order to cope with her religious principles and the lack of guidance she found in the bible, Susan was strict with certain aspects with the IVF procedure. There was little she could do about taking the drugs and all that they would do to her body – such abuse felt harsh and unnatural – but there was only one way and that was all there was to it. When it came to fertilisation she felt that she could have some control over the life she so scientifically agreed to plan and destroy. She sought the advice of her church and a kind man told her that she should not be worried about discarding embryos as God would surely not meet her at the gates with those "murdered" offspring with vengeance and disapproval.

Susan could not agree. It was still a life she had chosen to create and then disregard. She could not do it. Especially when her heart had been so touched by all the thousands of children in existence that needed a home and whom she wanted to help. She couldn't help but feel it was wrong to create yet more life, let alone discard an embryo so coldly. But she was a wife and had to compromise with her husband, since this was not all about her, and she was not yet certain of God's plan. She knew it was not fair on Mark or their children, however acquired, to insist on her own beliefs. They had to decide this as a married couple.

The decision to only fertilise two eggs haunted her throughout the entire IVF cycle and made her doubt her decision every step of the way. Placing only two eggs amongst the sperm was playing high stakes - people put lots more than that together and still only a few fertilise. While Susan knew this decision was not for everyone, she felt certain it was right for them and had felt that all the praying she had done had backed this decision up. They removed seven eggs in total: two were no good, two were average and three were good. They used ICSI on two of the good eggs. The staff constantly reminded her of the limited chance of success she should expect from such a decision – they found it hard to relate to. As they waited for the results of the fertilisation Susan questioned herself and what she was putting Mark through by being so rigid. Certain comments from friends didn't help either.

"What are you doing? The cost? The chances of success—?"

Susan was in tears and increasingly became despondent and uncertain. Call it luck of the draw, call it God blessing them for being so considerate or just simply something that was meant to be but both eggs fertilised. Susan received a phone call while having her bedroom carpet fitted to say that both were doing well. It took all her strength not to cry in front of the carpet fitter. They were implanted and the long wait began. They went on holiday to the Lake District on the day of implantation. Mark had wanted to spend the two weeks peacefully waiting to do the pregnancy test and was disappointed that the cottage they had rented had noisy people above them and they were unable to change cottages. As week two began so did the problems: Susan was admitted to hospital with OHSS (Ovarian Hyper-Stimulation Syndrome).

Her ovaries were filled with fluid and her abdomen was so bloated that she looked 6 months pregnant and could hardly walk. Mark spent every day with her at the hospital before taking the thirty minute journey back to the cottage and sleeping alone. He was gutted, felt terrible that they hadn't been able to spend time together and felt robbed of a holiday, but he had little time to think about it and was more worried about his wife. Some staff at the hospital were saying that it was impossible to tell whether or not she was pregnant because her hormones were all over the place, an affect of the IVF drugs, and with the water being retained in her ovaries they could not be sure. However, other staff were certain that she showed signs of pregnancy and they were excited, playfully displaying this every now and then. Mark refused to get his hopes up. He was a pessimist by nature and preferred to look at the worst case scenario, he felt this was an easier way of coping with disappointing results. He was desperate to know. It was ironic how many pregnancy tests they had done over the years, even purchasing multipacks and special offers, and yet now they couldn't do one. They had to wait a painfully long six weeks to have an internal scan before they knew whether or not they were still pregnant.

"Oh yes," said the obstetrician as he rummaged around internally as if he were looking for Jacobs cream crackers in the pantry. "Twin one is fine."

Susan burst out crying: she had just learned that not only was she pregnant but had twins. She shook with emotion and the obstetrician told her off and asked her to be still as she was making it difficult for him to scan her. Quite unintentionally, she ignored him. He had no idea that they hadn't done a pregnancy test and was genuinely shocked that this was the first they knew they were pregnant – at six weeks. It amused Mark immensely. All in all, they had about fourteen visits to the hospital to complete their IVF and it had been hard work. Mark was grateful that his manager was understanding of his last minute trips and felt blessed that he worked in such a supportive company.

They tried to eat in Wagga mamas, Wimbledon, calling and texting family members to let them know. Everyone was more excited than Mark, forever the pessimist, still preparing himself for the worst. Part of him felt that they were in the wrong by playing God; that this was unnatural and he didn't think that it would work. It wasn't just his gut feeling - he had seen copious amounts of scientific evidence stating that it was highly unlikely to work. He refused to get excited. Susan insisted on hiding from people who didn't know, blatantly aware that her stomach was still so swollen that she looked pregnant, and terrified that people would ask if she was. What would she tell them?

Her pregnancy was horrendous and the worst thing she had experienced.

"There was nothing lovely about it," Susan recalls. "Nothing!"

She hated everything about pregnancy and how she felt. It worried her that she felt no bond towards her unborn babies and it was nothing but a mere burden which introduced her to terrible indigestion and migraines. They had a couple of emergency visits to the hospital, who were excellent, and they monitored her well. Mark remembers little about the pregnancy.

"It's strange," he recalls. "I remember almost every difficult and painful stage of the IVF and fluid retention, which was a lot shorter in length, but cannot recall much of the entire pregnancy except how big Susan was and how difficult her day working in a primary school and bending over small children and sitting on little chairs must have been."

When she was thirty four weeks pregnant she started to feel better and even sat pondering one day upon how good she felt. She was certain she would go full term now; she had never felt this good. That evening she had a pain which refused to go away. It felt like an arm or an elbow digging into her and caused her great discomfort. She rang the hospital and they told her to just take some paracetamol. She did – it changed nothing. Susan wasn't feeling right. It was six weeks before the due date and something was wrong. They went to house group, with their local group of friends from church, and Mark even stopped to pick up a new guitar amp before they went to bed. When Susan was feeling increasingly uncomfortable he took her into hospital, at about 01:00, and she was monitored. They soon realised that she was having contractions and was dilated. They still, at this point, did not think the twins were coming – it was too early – so Mark went home at 05:00, had a short sleep, and then went to work as usual.

He was surprised when Susan called him to say they were going to be born that day and he needed to get there – the twins were breech and she was to have a caesarean. He cycled to the hospital as fast as his wobbling legs and stunned mind could take him as he forced himself to be calm, thinking about the practicalities: how could he take paternity leave now? What if they moved her to a different hospital since their local one was so full? He wouldn't be able to cycle there. He worried about the logistics as he cycled like a maniac.

He received another call from Susan.

"Hurry up, it's happening, I'm talking with the anaesthetist."

"The anaesthetist was called Sunny. He had the gift of the gab and made you feel that he was an expert and very capable with what he was doing. He made us feel very relaxed. He is not the sort of person you meet and forget," Mark explains.

Mark faced Susan as she had the epidural in her back and it pained him to watch. Once more, he realised how brave she was and she took it "like a trooper". He was just relieved that she had a caesarean because he couldn't have born to watch her in pain while giving birth naturally.

"We are very close, you see, and I couldn't bear to watch her go through that especially after all that she had been through," he sighs.

"Oh, nice contractions, they are going well," said the nurse somewhat indifferently. "You're already two centimetres dilated."

The twins were six weeks early but Susan wasn't worried. She had her faith and they were twins after all – this was to be expected. Initially, they said that she couldn't have them there because they would be premature and needed special attention and they were too busy to take her on but they became more concerned about her giving birth during an ambulance drive so made room. They were in a clinical environment with numerous amounts of strangers around them. Susan kept feeling sick and was given anti-sickness drugs. Mark's first thought upon seeing the twins was more of relief than anything else because the twins and his wife were OK. When they told him to come over and see the baby, to see what sex it was, Mark felt special – despite all the strangers - it was he, the father, the actual father, who would declare the sex of his child to Susan. This was the fondest memory he had.

"It's a boy," he smiled proudly.

Susan recollects hearing Daniel crying and vaguely realising that this was her baby crying, not just any baby, but her very own. It was surreal.

"It's another boy," Mark declares even more excitedly, waving his arms about. He was ecstatic at having two boys.

Everyone in the room laughed when Thomas piddled all over the floor as he was being lifted to the scales and it was a surprisingly warm moment. They took some wonderful photos of them all together before they were whisked away into care.

"It felt weird that they were then taken away into care when I had only just laid eyes upon them," Mark told me. "I had only just seen them and there was no bond and no withdrawal because I had only just met them – it was very surreal."

Mark, not usually such an emotional person, was overwhelmed and mesmerised at the sight of his twin boys, Daniel 3.15lb and Thomas 3.14 lb, and guarded them dearly. Susan was not allowed to see them because she had lost too much blood – this devastated her. But the next morning a kind nurse, shocked that she had not seen them, put her in a wheelchair and took her to them. The tubes didn't faze her at all, she barely noticed them since she had seen her cousin's twenty six week old twins in hospital previously – this was nothing in comparison. All her concerns about the lack of bond disappeared as she set eyes upon her boys and felt the immense love that arose from within.

Mark took photos and brought them down for Susan to see. He felt sorry that she wasn't able to go up herself and was relieved when he could take her up in her wheelchair. They spent a peculiar week in the hospital: no sleep at night, he went to work during the day, and despite his exhaustion, was able to run on sheer excitement and adrenaline. When Susan was really tired, the nurses took the boys away overnight and watched them in the nursery, allowing her to get some sleep. Susan still found it hard to sleep with other visitors not leaving until really late; people on mobile phones, lights going on and off, nurse visits bringing pills.

Girl's names had been easier to choose but they had struggled with boy's. In fact, they were calling them twin one and twin two for so long that the doctor threatened to name them himself if they didn't get a move on. Daniel was often dressed in green; it became his colour, while Thomas was blue. It was immediately obvious how dissimilar they were. They were there all week and were finally discharged at 22:00. Mark remembers, gravely, that it was raining and it was the scariest journey of his life.

"I drove so slowly and felt so very alone with all this responsibility in the car. It was scary," he says, shaking his head as he remembers.

It was a great relief to both of them to be going home and have some control over their sleep. Or so they thought.

They were plunged straight into it: twelve feeds per night, an amount that shocked them both to their core. They soon got into a system of feeding one each but it didn't work very well because you would always hear the other one wake up so neither of them slept. Mark found that even making the formula was a challenge: the stress to get it right in the middle of the night under the pressure of a crying and hungry baby was a lot to suddenly take on. It wasn't long before they were actually hallucinating with sleep deprivation.

"I would roll over onto one of the twins and squash them," Mark recalls tragically, "only realising that they were in their cot and I had imagined it. Or Susan asked if I had fed Thomas and I confirmed that I had – but I hadn't – I'd imagined that too! It was terrifying."

Mark had a close shave when his bike hit a car on his way to work one day and it was a wakeup call for him. He thought he had broken his leg and limped to work and proudly showed me the scars still visible on his leg and elbow. He was in shock and sent home from work. He slept on the sofa he was so exhausted.

"I couldn't even drive properly," he remembers. "I was scared of running people over when I was in a mad rush and not seeing pedestrians and I couldn't get clutch control at all. All the simple and basic things in life just became incredibly difficult to do. I reckon that during those first six months my judgement was severely impaired."

The health visitors didn't help either: unable to give good advice and instead passing on opinions as if they were fact. This was very confusing and Mark didn't like them. They warned him not to use the microwavable steriliser they had purchased, making him feel like a bad person for thinking of such a thing, and forcing him to go out and buy an electric one – which broke. Eventually, they used the microwave one and found it much easier and less time consuming.

"It's just difficult, as a new parent, to get used to what is right and wrong," Mark muses. "You aren't sure, you want advice and help but I hated the fact that they used scare tactics when voicing their opinions or recommendations, which might not suit us, as if it were fact and the only way. Life was much easier when we stopped seeing them."

Daniel was not well at first and developed a serious case of acid reflux. There was puke everywhere, constantly, and the smell lingered in the house for months no matter how often everything was washed.

"It's a smell that will remain with us for a long time," Susan cringes.

They had to raise his cot so high that they would find him crumpled at the bottom in the morning covered in puke. He didn't gain weight for the first three months despite the twelve feeds per night. Mark found work increasingly difficult with the sleep-deprivation kicking in so Susan had to take on the nights and all the feeds alone. The twins refused to sleep through the night no matter how hard she tried to encourage it.

"With hindsight," Susan smiles, "I wish I had just woken them up and fed them."

The sleep deprivation consumed their lives and was incredibly difficult to bear. Susan refused to believe or resented the fact that other children slept through from only a few weeks old. Her boys refused to sleep through the night for nine months – an incredibly long time for a sleep-deprived parent. The first night they actually slept through was the first of January. Susan laughs with joy as she proclaims it was the twins New Year resolution. Eventually, they didn't feel as if they could cope any longer and Mark called his parents: they were over in a shot. They looked after the children and let Mark and Susan catch up on sleep during the day. When Mark was feeling better he would take the children out for two and three hour walks to let Susan sleep.

"Susan is the sort of person who always needs a lot of sleep so I knew how hard this was on her. I wanted to give her that time and space."

He would sit in the park watching football all afternoon with them sleeping on and off in their pram. He even purchased Susan a pass for Nirvana spa and, when the twins were six months old, she had her first day off.

"It was the worst day of my life," Mark recalls. "It was such a hard day for me and it gave me a snapshot of what Susan's week must be like. I felt really bad for her. They were so hard to juggle."

The latest Mark gets home is 17:45 and he considers himself a hands on father. He does nappies, bath time every evening, he spends time with them before work, he cleans all the bottles daily and does almost all of the housework – he is very dedicated – even taking them out at the weekends to give Susan a break (albeit often to just do chores!). Susan's problems in pregnancy did not leave her after the birth. A few months after the boys were born she awoke in the middle of the night with the most excruciating pain in her chest. It took her breath away. Having known a friend who had suffered a serious problem after a caesarean, she was scared the same thing had happened to her. The pain was how she imagined child birth must be – it was that bad. Concerned, she called an ambulance. However, with sleep-deprivation ruling their lives, she was actually more concerned with the ambulance waking up the boys and urged them to be quiet. She was given some gas and air before passing out on the lounge floor. She was much better afterwards as the paramedic calmly explained that she had indigestion. She was in denial: it was far too painful to be that.

"Honestly, it's indigestion," the paramedic explained kindly.

Having to explain to the concerned neighbours the next day that it was merely indigestion was incredibly embarrassing but she had to put their minds at ease that the boys were fine. It has not left her since. Each devastatingly painful episode of indigestion lasts between an hour and an hour and a half. She has to go on all fours to relive the pain for the entire time and cannot breathe properly. She has to do this while tending to the needs of her twin boys. In addition, she continues to take copious amounts of medication for the migraines that become so bad she loses her sight temporarily. It's hardly surprising that Susan never wishes to get pregnant again. While Susan did not enjoy her pregnancy, or the IVF, she has no regrets but will not choose to do either again. She feels no need or desire to have any more children but hopes to still adopt when the twins are older. Mark confesses to having one hour on a Monday where he plays football and that is his "me" time. Susan is too tired and chooses to go to bed early instead of taking on any other activities for herself.

"I find it ironic," he says, "that before I became a dad I was always on the go and always had to be achieving something. Never, in a million years, did I think I would be content to spend the day in the house and garden – let alone a whole weekend – I was never like that."

They are organised enough to get the boys to bed, cook tea and sit down by 19:45 to eat and watch TV or talk about things that have to be done, such as insurance renewals.

"My greatest challenge," Mark humbly admits. "Is trying to enjoy now and the time I have with them at this age instead of thinking about the future and how I will like it when they can do more grown up things. I need to gain more patience, that is always a challenge with me, and stop thinking about the future."

"How would you sum up fatherhood?" I ask.

He thinks about it for a while. "Exhausting," he says rolling his eyes. "Constantly exhausting. I used to have such high standards about things such as cleanliness and all my expectations have been lowered. I couldn't stand a messy or dirty house but now I just don't care as much."

Mark strongly believes that the boys are miracles and God has been faithful to them, and he feels fortunate.

"It's a privilege and a great responsibility," he says. "But we wouldn't have survived without all the support we have received."

There are two sets of people Mark is particularly grateful to: their parents, particularly his own who are younger and more able and were there in a nano-second whenever they were called for days at a time. And the church: they did a rota of meals and took turns cooking meals each night for them and left it on their doorstep.

"We just couldn't have done it without that support. We have had fairly incredible support over the last eighteen months." He visibly shudders. "We just couldn't have done it without them - we could not have survived."

Chapter 10 - Callously Deserted

The Friday before mother's day James emailed me from work to say that he would be home late. Alarm bells rang: he wasn't the sort of man who worked late often, particularly on a Friday, and he would normally call. I watched the clock. In a decade he had never before been home later than seven thirty. By nine o'clock I was worried. By ten o'clock I knew he was with someone. With a sinking heart I went to bed to wait it out. A week earlier we had gone to bed, as usual, and not for the first time he asked me to have sex.

"I need sex soon," he said coldly, staring up at the ceiling.

It had been a while, months to be honest, since the weekly dates had proved such a disaster and such statements like this was the only form of affection he showed me. I resented the lack of romance or effort and I was constantly exhausted. Our relationship was based on avoidance because his spite continued and far from turned me on.

"Thanks for telling me, I appreciate the effort," I replied in a similar cold tone and turned my back on him. I felt cheap and worthless.

I had organised more evenings out with him than any couple I knew and all I needed was a little bit more than such a statement last thing at night. He had sabotaged every night out, arguing or moaning, and nothing good had come of them. During the last month I hadn't arranged a night out and had given up trying. The twins were fourteen months old. He finally came home at midnight and I pretended to be asleep as he snuck into bed. He had only two friends from university, who were not local, and he met them once or twice a year at best. Over the weekend he acted odd, could not make eye contact and looked away whenever I looked at him. I kept busy with the twins and decided whether to confront him or not. We had mother's day lunch booked with his mum and his cousin who was visiting from Canada with her newborn. It was my second mother's day and once again I got nothing – it hurt. We were civil. When we got home, I asked him if he had anything to say to me, but he merely shook his head and walked away. I waited until he came home from work the next day and calmly asked again. He poured me a large glass of wine and gave me that look.

"I don't love you in the same way that I used to," he said, before burying his head in his hands.

I down the glass of wine and pour another, crying harder than ever before. I was drowning in wine and rejection. It didn't matter that he had treated me terrible since I became a mother – I loved him – I adored him and I never, in a million years, expected this. I thought I would have to forgive an affair not be abandoned. Drunk and emotional, I hysterically ramble certain things at him while he remains his normal introvert and silent self as he watches me unfold.

"I wouldn't love me either; look at the state of me!" I scream. "I'm nothing like the woman I used to be. I'm broken! I'm fat! I'm ugly and I'm a horrible person!"

I was in shock. I packed some bags and the next morning I took the children and stayed with my sister for the week. I was numb. Was he really going to leave me or say something wonderful when I returned? I was distracted with all the activities while at my sisters and numbly got through the week. Friday evening, on the two hour drive home, I was expecting – hoping - for some sort of a declaration of love and an apology. I was disappointed. He remained unchanged in his resolve. I could not believe that he was willing to give up everything just to get away from me and it hurt acutely. He planned to move in with his brother but they had guests staying over the weekend so he had to wait until Monday. He was snappy, impatient and horrible to me and the children all day Saturday. His mum was coming up to see him, having heard the news, and I insisted she could not come to the house – I couldn't bear to see her and blamed her for the tension she had put on us since the twins were born. They went out to dinner and she apparently gave him a hard time about leaving me and the children, which will undoubtedly mortify her publically and that was all she cared about, and yet I desperately hoped she succeeded at turning him around.

I learned how forceful she was towards him upon his return when he takes it out on me and am certain he remained silent in front of his mother. He must despise me immensely and it hurts. I could not bear the hate I could see in the eyes that used to show adoration – how that look had changed. I was too hurt to stand up for myself and just took the abuse until I burst out crying and ran into my bed. I sobbed all through the night, muffling as much of the noise as I could in the pillow, not wanting him or the children to hear me. I was too loud and knew he could hear. I felt very ashamed. I should be stronger.

By the morning I was stronger. I had a little bit of pride still in me somewhere and the shame had turned into immense anger. When he apologised for how he had treated me, with all his usual lack of sincerity, I declare that it wasn't good enough.

"I will not stand for you treating me like this ever again. It would break my heart if Beth allowed a man to treat her so disrespectfully and I have to set an example. Get out now. Right now!" I said steadily and with determination.

"No! I can't go until tomorrow, you'll just have to tolerate me one more day," he replied nastily.

"No I don't," I said with strength I never knew I had. "You have made your feelings clear and I will not take this from you any longer. Get your things and go now!"

"Where to? Where am I supposed to stay? We're broke, we have no money!"

"That is not my problem and for the record, we are going to be a lot more bloody broke from now on! Just get out. I don't care if you sleep in the car overnight! I'm not having you here treating me like this in front of the children. You've made your choice."

He was furious. He banged all the doors and stomped about the house as he packed. I hurt inside but fury had set in. He crept out of the house without saying goodbye while I sat holding hands with my Reverend in the lounge who had been hoping that James would sit and talk to him, either alone or with me, but James had refused to even acknowledge his presence and ignored us completely. He just left. I was disappointed that both the Reverend and my mother-in-law couldn't stop him. I refused to beg or try and part of me just gave up on him.

My Reverend was the only selfless person I knew.

We had a holiday booked at Centre Parks in less than two weeks, something I hoped would help our relationship, as it did last year, but he had no intention of going with me. My life had just dramatically altered course. I loved him. I hated him. I was hurt. I was angry. I was more furious that he would leave the children and was more concerned about the effect of that than how he felt about me – how could he do that to his children! I was in shock. I didn't feel the same about him either, which was normal and what I expected given the circumstances, but it never crossed my mind to split up. Once the twins were older and less dependent it got easier and that was when we were supposed to re-establish our life. I married a man who I thought would stand by my side forever. I never saw this coming. I never thought he would leave me. I simply could not believe it.

He stayed at the house for the week that I was away in Centre Parks so he could have time to think and housesit the cat and chickens for me. I took my pregnant niece and a friend with her toddler. I learned that my friend wanted another baby and was an emotional wreck because she hadn't fallen pregnant in the four months she had been trying. She threw a tantrum, burst out crying and packed and left on the second day.

"I just cannot be around a pregnant woman right now!" she declared tearfully.

My niece felt terrible and hid in her bedroom and I just couldn't relate to this friend of mine: four months of trying was nothing compared to the year's most people suffered especially since she already had a toddler. She was obviously depressed but I was lacking in sympathy. Her problems seemed trivial compared to mine which I later regretted thinking but couldn't help it at the time and I was annoyed with her because I needed her friendship. My niece and I got through the rest of the holiday and I tried to be good company for her. It was not great, my back was terrible now I lack the time to do yoga to keep it strong, and as a result my ankles were so weak they gave way under me and I fell, for no reason at all, while carrying my daughter in a back carrier. Fortunately I didn't land on her and only lose skin from my hands and knees but it was worrying. My ankle was swollen and I had to limp back to the villa with one twin still on my back while pushing the other in a trike. I wanted to burst out crying but had to consider the twins and how they would feel if I cried constantly.

We returned home and I focused on doing the laundry on the Saturday while my niece was still around to watch the children. I thought nothing of the pink knickers I pulled out of the laundry and handed to my niece.

"They aint mine!" she said turning her nose up in disgust.

"Are you sure?" I frown.

"Like!" Which I interpreted as teenage Birmingham for, "Yes, I'm sure, they're not my type."

I assumed they belonged to my friend and put them in the pile with her few forgotten toys and clothes. I thought nothing more of it until two weeks later when she visits and tells me that they aren't hers either. Our eyes lock and realisation sets in. I could see she felt sorry for me. The only laundry had been what I returned with from the holiday and the spare bed he had slept in. He denies bringing anyone back to my house.

The children were affected and people started commenting on how unusually reserved they were at play groups. They were not their normal outgoing selves and were whiny, clingy and refusing to leave my side: it broke my heart. He hadn't just left me he had left them and they deserved better. He had just made my life incredibly hard. I had to do everything on my own and it was impossible with one year old twins, a dog, a cat, tropical fish and chickens. Something had to go. I couldn't sleep and it didn't help when the dog woke me at four in the morning because a fox was in the garden: I'd forgotten to lock the chicken's up and the fox had killed them all. I was slowly losing everything but at least that was one less chore.

The children kept coming into my bed and I wondered which of us craved the cuddles the most. I was spending too much time at the gym and putting the twins in the crèche. I sat numb and blank in the Jacuzzi and steam room or did a twenty minute meditation at the side of the pool with my iPod. I had no energy or motivation to work out. I fell asleep one day and awoke myself with the most horrendous man-like snoring to find a group of about fifteen women doing aqua-aerobics laughing at me. They made comments such as, "you must have needed that," nodding at the band on my wrist declaring that I had children in the crèche. It was so embarrassing.

I had no social life, missed adult conversation, and the phone never rang. Bitterness towards my friends consumes me – where have they all ran to and why? I was always inviting them here but they didn't come anymore and I received no invites in return. I distrusted everyone now. I realised that an uncommitted friend, one who never calls or visits when you clearly needed them, was worse than no friend – they just reinforced my sense of rejection and failure – it shocked me. I was lucky that the local group had just started a parenting course that could keep me occupied. They played with the children while we drank coffee and chatted about discipline, reward charts and child development. It was nice to be able to talk about it and focus on what to do. I kept busy, the evenings were painfully long, lonely and tedious with so much housework and I felt utterly depressed. I was too extrovert and sociable to handle such isolation. Sometimes I was so tired I forgot that I had tidied up and it was a lovely surprise waking up to a clean house.

I tried not to indulge myself in sorrow, self-pity or depression because the twins deserved a better mother than that but I was fighting a losing battle with no support. I should be enjoying this time with them and dwell on what it should be like. I blow at the slightest thing and feel utterly ashamed as a mother. Since being on anti-depressants I noticed that my depression was more hormonal because even the anti-depressants could not stop the severe blackout I entered during my cycle. I plunged into darkness and burst into excessive bouts of tears or anger. When I cried, it felt as if the whole world was caving in on me and everything was so much worse than it was. Or I was simply numb and unresponsive.

It was taking every ounce of willpower to not shout at the children constantly. My immune system was terrible and I'd been constantly ill since having the twins and I'm moody as hell when I'm ill. It had been three months since James walked out on me and I found him really unpleasant. The twins second birthday party was awkward and I had to ask for James three times, holding back my annoyance, in order to get a family picture with the cake. I didn't know what was the best thing to do and stuck with what I would do normally. I wondered how I was going to explain all this to them later on. Without children, I would have been miserable, with children, their father was miserable – what do I tell them so that they feel secure and happy within themselves? How do I encourage them to respect their father when I had no respect for him as a man, husband or father at all? Such thoughts weigh heavily on me and left me with no answers.

A friend talks me into joining an on line dating agency and I had a fling with a local divorced man, just two dates, in an attempt to boost my ego. I learned how easy it was to pull regardless of my body. However, it also made me feel bad because I was now just seen as easy meat, desperate and nothing more than a shag. This was the world I had entered.

A long-term friend finally returns my calls to ask how I am. Upon hearing about the fling, and ignoring the fact that I knew him a few weeks before inviting him round, which I only did in the end after too much wine and a huge argument with James, she began to lecture me. I was being irresponsible, putting my children at risk and not being a good mother. I tried to explain that since I had no family or friends to visit me, no babysitters and no ability to leave the house once the children were in bed, I was left in a very lonely and difficult situation and the very last thing I needed right now was to be called a bad mother. I knew how depressed I was, still had thoughts that the children would be better off without me, and was desperately trying to hold myself together. She called me naive, selfish and irresponsible. I was furious and knew that I did not need a friend to judge me so harshly and make me feel bad about myself under the current situation. She hadn't even visited me in the three months since James left, nor been on the end of the phone, but now called to parent me. She said we should just agree to disagree but what bothered me was the tone with which the disapproval was delivered.

"I am their Godmother and have to look out for the children when you are clearly not. I care about them and you are obviously not putting them first—" she tells me in a condescending tone.

I was surprised and had never been spoken to like this, especially from her, and I almost burst into tears. Her role as Godparent was to guide my children spiritually not lecture me on my parenting skills and put me down. I did everything for the twins and they knew nothing of this brief fling. I was not the one who walked out and left - I stayed here meeting their every need and where were my friends? No one was there for me. I had given this friend my car, when she totalled her vehicle and could not afford another, I had been there when her boyfriend left her with a child and when her second lover treated her like dirt. I kept silent as I watched her put her new boyfriend before her son, minding my own business because I knew it wouldn't last for long and, most importantly, was none of my business. I felt completely let down.

I was fortunate that my GP, upon hearing my black thoughts, had signed me up for a CBT (cognitive behaviour therapy) course in self-esteem building and the ten weeks talking with a nurse was giving me a lot of emotional strength. I often believe that without this course, this friend's words would have led me to suicide. I would always be grateful to my GP and have never spoken to this friend of fifteen years since. I was obviously not myself at the time and this was not the sort of treatment I needed. She never apologised or showed any interest in being in our lives since.

Saturday was my first night without them, since they were born, and they were staying overnight with James at his parent's house, ninety minutes drive away, while they were in France. I didn't handle it well. I was too worried about their well-being. I spent all day and evening lying on the sofa severely depressed and crying a lot. I was also having horrendous side-effects from coming off the anti-depressants too early because they're not helping anymore and made it hard to get up in the mornings. I was bound to be depressed under the circumstances and pills weren't going to bring him back all happy and full of love. They're not helping because they couldn't change my life.

I was scared of James flipping and doing something dangerous and taking the children away from me. It was men who bury their depression who suddenly go crazy and my mind raced with thoughts of him killing the children and then himself. Such a case had recently been on the news. I was terrified that I wouldn't see the twins again. It was a horrible position to be in; wanting the children to have time with their father and knowing he was unable to cope and may snap, feeling protective and fearful while trying to do the right thing. I was just glad they came home to me. I could not believe how much James and I had deteriorated. We used to be able to talk and understand each other but now we end up not listening and just being spiteful. I hadn't been sleeping, which didn't help. There was too much to do and the children had been sick. I'll never forgive him. He hadn't even given it a chance – I could easily end up hating him.

I'd aged a lot in the last year; I saw it in my face as the mirror winced from my reflection. I washed my hair but brushed it only once or twice a week, the rest of the time it was pulled back into a frizzy and untidy bun. The saying "there isn't enough hours in the day" had never rang more true. I was still fat and felt hopeless about doing a thing to change myself. The day began at five and ended at ten, on a good day, or normally midnight. I never got a cup of tea hot or sat for ten minutes. This was just covering the basics and excluded my hygiene. I had never worked so hard and it was the most unrewarding, tedious of chores that I found the hardest. Just as I finished, it was time to start the same thing all over again. The children trashed a room as soon as it was cleaned. I couldn't sleep. No matter what I cut back on it didn't seem to get easier. I was screaming and shouting at the children far too often.

I went to the job centre with the children and found out what my rights and options were. I had never sought benefits before, had worked since the age of eight in my parent's hotel and never been anything less than independent. It was alien to me, I loathed going and didn't fit in with the type of people cursing around me. The twins were playing up and I was nervous of them being around some of the more volatile people obviously on something. Nothing was straight forward and there were no set answers. I gathered enough information, signed up for Income Support explaining that my children had just lost their father and they were not losing me to be raised by a stranger. I felt so sick I vomited in the car park on my way out. Copious amounts of phone calls and paper work followed. No one would give me straight answers so I had to dig hard and figure it all out with two screaming children and no time on my hands. The phone was glued to my ear and my heart raced. I didn't yet know what he planned to do and had arranged to see a solicitor and file for divorce – I needed to know where we stood financially and secure the children's future.

   I had little faith that a man who left his children when they were only one, with very little bonding, would stay around for the long haul. I was more worried about him meeting another woman or staying with the one he was seeing and her moaning about how much money he gave to us – I always thought ahead and knew he would be difficult if either of us moved on. It took weeks of persistent phone calls, letters and forms to gather an idea of where I stood. I had many tearful phone calls with James. The worst fear was if he refused to cover the mortgage and what would happen to the house. I rang a few mortgage companies, gave them a false name and my details and learned that unless I had been in work for a number of months I stood no chance of getting the mortgage renewed – it went on my status – not his or joint - and, according to three banks, he now had no motivation to cover the mortgage because he was not resident here. They deemed the fact that his children resided here as irrelevant.

   We were forced to remortgage for a fixed five years, losing a few thousand pounds off the equity in the process, while pretending we were still together. It secured the house temporarily. I should be earning by then and remortgage on my own merit. If he refused to cover the mortgage, which he wasn't legally obliged to do, I would lose the house but the equity in it wasn't enough to buy anything outright in a nice area, and exempted me from social housing I'd rather not need or have anyhow. I felt sick to the core. I would have to lose all my equity on rented accommodation before I qualified for social housing leaving me in my forties, off the property ladder, moving the children two or four times in their early years – more disruption – and end up financially where I was after university. I was horror struck. My world had just fallen apart and I could lose everything I had spent the past twenty years building up. It was all too much for me to bear. My Birthday came and went without me realising until I got a couple of cards in the post – not my usual forty or more – thanks friends. Everyone was obviously upset with me and disliked or blamed me somehow and I felt desperately hurt and resentful because it seemed so unfair. I was the one who stayed.

The twin's behaviour was worse after seeing their dad and grandparents and it filled me with hate: I shouldn't have to give my children up like this and suffer such behaviour upon their return. I tried to understand that this was normal, to a degree, and be careful not to blame everything on my circumstances – many of the mum's said how naughty the children were after visiting grandparents or a holiday - I just had to face it weekly. They didn't understand what was going on, their dad had become intermittent and withdrawn, his behaviour was strange and forced, their grandparents disappeared for weeks on end, their mum was suddenly shouting like a Banshee, was too tired and busy to play with them in the way they were used to and even seemed to dislike having them around most of the time. How were they supposed to understand all this at their age? I was eating junk food and drinking too much wine to get extra energy for the evening's workload and numb the emotional pain. Half a bottle of wine and I'd clean the kitchen, make a dinner for tomorrow, vacuum and mop: a full bottle and I would get the ironing done too. It may get the chores done but the guilt at being an irresponsible mother ate away at me and deepened my depression, especially when binge drinking parents or those who drink alone were mentioned on BBC Breakfast.

I had been incredibly selfish since James left because all I thought about was myself, the space and break I needed, how much I had to do, how much I'd lost and how tired I was. I didn't want to be like this but seemed powerless to engage with my children like I used to. I had been sticking the TV on far too much and putting the twins in the crèche almost daily while I swam. I'd withdrawn from the twins and felt guilty; the circumstances, depression and the overwhelming workload had sent me into a state of shock. After a few weeks of this I drafted out a schedule and planned my week better, ensuring I cut down at the gym, spent quality time with them, interacted more throughout each day and showed them how much I loved them. The Banshee had to go. I was scared because a big part of me didn't want to be here. It was not the children I wanted to leave but the house and chores – I had serious cabin fever and hated being housebound. I loved them but I could not stand this hard life all alone.

I showed the twins how to pop bubble wrap but their fingers were too little to do it. Undeterred, I placed it on the floor and showed them how to dig their big toe in and pop it that way. BANG! Howls of laughter filled the room. It just saddened me when we had a laughing moment like this because they were so rare when they should be regular occurrences. I hated him. I would never forgive him for sending me into emotional turmoil so soon after having the twins. The bastard! I resentfully watched other new mothers relishing their new status and noticed that only a few, like me, seemed to be struggling.

Divorce was easier to understand than Income Support but trying to tie down what I needed covered and what would interfere with my Income Support status was proving hard to ascertain. It took almost a month to get confirmation that if he paid me money towards the mortgage or gas and electric then it was considered as indirect income and I lost my benefits. However, if he paid the mortgage direct it was not taken into account – such a trivial thing could have a huge effect on my finances. It was better for him to pay the mortgage direct than give me spouse maintenance. Having earned more than James and suddenly being on benefits just because I chose to stay home with my children was soul destroying and I pushed my selfish pride aside for the sake of the children. I knew this was the best thing for them right now, to have my love and attention. Going back to work would also leave me worse off financially with the costs of childcare and it wasn't a viable option. Even if I miraculously found an IT job that paid highly, given the circumstances, it would have destroyed my children even though I would have been much happier at work and earning again. They wouldn't have seen me much so I wouldn't really have been happier – I knew this.

A teenager moved in with me temporarily during the summer holidays as an English au pair and helped me with the children while I sorted out all the paperwork and financials. I worked hard to keep the divorce amicable in order to get the best response from James. I had met a few divorced women lately and their stories had not been nice. The nastiness and spite that can go on was alarming because it was the children who suffered. I had the rest of my life to work with James and knew how important it was to not let the divorce get out of control and turn sour. It was bad enough when the man walks out on you but if he was violent or played games and fought for every penny then it was even harder. If the woman turned revengeful and used the children then it was a blood-bath.

One woman told me how her husband sold the house from under her nose while she was having chemotherapy in hospital, having learned she had cancer during her divorce, and he had been the one to initially walk out. She had to sleep on a friend's sofa and fortunately pulled through - she was understandably very bitter. My own sister had been trying to seal her divorce for three years and he was fighting for just a few grand, refusing to compromise, purposefully lost his job to avoid CSA payments for his three children and it was forcing the children involved to take sides. I was shocked and appalled that CSA legally ended when a child was only a teenager and so many fathers used this as an excuse to stop contributing towards their keep. They blank their minds to housing costs, education, car, commuting for an apprenticeship or job at an age when the teenager most needed financial support – it opened my eyes to something I had never before considered and my fear of the future was overwhelming. I couldn't find a nice divorce story anywhere and some sounded like horror movies.

The au pair was lovely and the twins took to her straight away. James was being amicable and giving me money towards childcare on top of the CSA. She would only be here for a few weeks before going to university but it gave me that space to sort everything out and get on top of everything. She was away at the weekends and I liked that. I learned about boarding school syndrome from the radio and looked it up – the inability to handle relationships and communicate emotions was exactly where James struggled – and I forwarded him the information. Apparently, more men were currently voicing their concerns about their life being ruined because they were raised from a young age by teachers, in boarding schools, and how it left them ill-equipped to handle real life situations outside of the workplace. They claimed they were emotionally stunted because they were not raised with a loving family and often ended up having issues with women that relate to being abandoned by their mothers.

I didn't really care – I was still having to get divorced – whatever the reason. While he admitted this was definitely something he could connect with it didn't help our situation. I was not sure if I wanted him to blame that and ask to come back or if I just wanted him to overcome his depression but it didn't get me anywhere. I went to boarding school too but much later, aged thirteen, and I could clearly understand how being raised by people unconnected to you would be a lot different than being raised by parents and sibling who thought you were special. When I told my parents I didn't want to board they let me come home daily. James never had that choice. I looked at my twins and knew which one would thrive and which one would struggle with the same scenario because Chris was far more sensitive than Beth. That was a need, certainly not a weakness, and James was just as sensitive. My brother-in-law coped a little bit better with boarding school so early on because he was more like me and Beth but he still, like his brother, has no respect for women.

He won't talk to me or say anything above "I don't love you in the same way." He was amicable and generous in the divorce and didn't want to see the children move home and lose the advantage of the superb schools in this area. He was doing everything for them and, at least financially, was putting them first. I felt as if he was buying us off, throwing money at us to help ease his guilt and get him freedom from parental responsibility, and me, but as long as the children were secure I didn't complain. Their future was all that mattered to me.

I swallowed all my hurt and the immense anger in order to have an amicable divorce. This deepened my depression, especially the suppressed anger, and I accepted that. I was only relieved that I repressed my anger and turned it on myself rather than lashing out – especially since my children were the ones around me all day long. I was glad to be the only one who suffered it. I didn't care how I felt. I had to protect my children. Part of me wished that I had left him during infertility and found someone who did want a family and not just me but then these exact two children wouldn't exist and they were too adorable to regret that. He was still very moody and snide, conversation was a continuous battle, and it took all my will power and vats of wine to bite my tongue and control my fist (dad should never have taught me to box!)

My collie dog died when I was a teenager and it broke my heart. I vowed that when I was older and had my own dog that I would breed her and keep a bitch of a bitch so that I always had a part of her when she passed away. I planned to breed Fudge and didn't want to lose that option just because I was alone. In fact, having no one else made it even more important to me. She was almost three so I should do it soon or lose the chance. I could also do with having some backup money in case there was a problem with the boiler or car since I was not earning anything. We had already paid for the stud and all her hip and elbow scoring, which cost over a thousand pounds, and it would have been a shame to waste that money. On the other hand, it could cost me money, would increase my daily workload to an almost impossible level and I might not be able to home all the puppies. I decided to go ahead.

I had the au pair here to help with the children and hopefully the first few weeks. As I watched the stud dog having his naughty way with my best friend all I could think of was how pregnancy was highly likely in just two or three well-timed ties. Was it that humans had fertility issues compared to dogs or that we only tended to breed a few of the best dogs so didn't tend to find fertility issues there? There was no need for an ovulation monitor with dogs; dates and the bitch flagging when she was ready were sufficient. It seemed unfair. I wanted to keep myself busy so I didn't have time to dwell upon the divorce proceedings and succumb to self-pity – keeping occupied distracted me from the dark turmoil bubbling away inside.

Chapter 11 - Michael and Fiona

Michael and Fiona are a brave, compassionate, incredibly romantic, loving and generous. Michael grew up in a large family, with two brothers and three sisters, he was in the middle, always surrounded by younger children, mostly in church, and this is what led him to become a youth worker. He grew up with a romantic notion towards marriage but with little desire to become a father and have children of his own. He tells me that he was quite an ugly child, which I find hard to believe with his boyish good looks and overwhelming charm, but this prevented him from having any relationships until he was about twenty one. He also had a strong desire to marry before he had sex, his girlfriend at the time wanted more, and three months into their relationship, he succumbed and they became intimate. He awoke the next morning terrified that she might be pregnant. The fear and guilt consumed him and he couldn't stop thinking about it. Fortunately, she was not, and within a year their relationship ended. It left him with a much clearer view of the type of relationship he wanted.

Being a very emotional person, he found the loss of the relationship very hard and he protected his heart dearly, he wouldn't date anyone again, instead choosing the safety of friendship to get to know a girl until he found "the ultimate one." He was at college when Fiona moved into his life. They were on the same course and Fiona frequently used his expertise to help her and pounded him with questions about theology. Fiona had a party in her small one bedroom flat and everyone was enjoying themselves while she hid in the kitchen. This was when Michael learned that she was incredibly awkward in front of people and, despite her love of socialising, often used the washing up as an excuse to avoid the crowd. Michael found her in the kitchen, refusing to mingle with her guests, and helped her feel more comfortable by helping her wash up. Fiona was consuming copious amounts of red wine and was grateful for his company. He understood her instantly and their friendship blossomed. Yet there was no expectation of a relationship forming above friendship for either of them, especially because Fiona, somewhat of a temptress, had eyes on someone else - Jake, who house-shared with Michael. Bonfire night confused Michael because he knew Fiona had a crush on Jake but he also felt that she was hitting on him when she wore his gloves to warm her freezing hands. She almost, at one point, held his hand too.

"Yeah, wearing gloves is a really big thing for a Christian boy and obviously means I'm after him!" Fiona laughs teasingly as Michael sits and blushes.

"She was also asking me probing questions about my past and girlfriends," Michael added. "She did it in a way that made me think that she was interested."

"I liked him," Fiona confesses. "But I was concerned that he was on the rebound because he still hadn't moved on from his last girlfriend."

Michael's birthday fell in November and he held a party. The house was heaving. Fiona had helped to decorate the house for his party but not for Michael's benefit, rather because Jake was going to be there too, and her crush was strong. Their entire year group were incredibly close and the party went well. At this point, they were starting to see each other as more than friends but neither of them wanted to take a risk and open up to the other. Happy Feet was showing on the cinema and Fiona desperately wanted to see it. Everyone was planning on going but Jake - who said he would rather have his eyeballs tattooed. Fiona lost her crush on him in that instant. Having penguins in the film made it her absolute favourite film – she is penguin mad - and how could she possibly like a man who didn't like Happy Feet? Michael was more than pleased. He had already had to witness, with distaste, her engagement to Anil, a Hindu who put his family before Fiona. Their wedding was set but Anil would not oppose his family who refused to accept the cultural difference between the engaged couple. It had taken a long time before Anil admitted this to Fiona and the relationship ended with her broken heart. She was disheartened with men and severely hurt. Her friendship with Michael remained safe and reassuring; she didn't want to lose that. Fiona got a new job and raced to Michael's house to tell him. It was at the same place he had just booked himself into as a youth worker. Now Michael was really nervous, his emotions were escalating and he was falling in love with her.

"If it weren't for Lent, we would never have got together," Fiona tells me excitedly. "I gave up chocolate and coffee and Michael gave up talking!"

Fiona took advantage of his silence. She has nineteen foster brothers and sisters and a father who suffered with depression. She adored her father. She hated sharing the news about her father's suicide, when she was only nineteen, which continues to haunt her. There was something else which bothered her: she had polycystic ovaries and was unlikely to be able to conceive. Whenever she told anyone about these things, she always felt disappointed or let down by their response. It had been bothering Fiona that Michael knew nothing of her secrets but with Michael being silent for lent, she could open up to him, knowing that he wasn't able to say anything that would upset her. Once Fiona opened up it all poured out. Michael showed little reaction and over the days she talked and talked and talked. Fiona sent an information pack to Michael about polycystic ovaries, which Michael believes was supposed to be a scare tactic to keep him away from her.

"But it didn't put me off at all," he smiles, putting his arm around her, "because she doesn't see herself in the same way that I or anyone else see's her."

Her polycystic ovaries give Fiona increased testosterone levels and her copious amount of dark body hair really upsets her. She had gone to India once, with Anil, and the women there were shocked at how hairy she was and wanted to wax her arms. They looked at her and treated her as if she were a freak of nature. Fiona became even more self-conscious about this and her embarrassment grew. She also had chronic Acne in her early teens so her self-esteem has always been very low.

"You don't seem unnaturally hairy to me," I laugh, since we are joking about it. "Mind you, that's probably because I'm so hairy anyway - my little sister calls me Chewbacca, that creature out of star wars, and I have to wax my moustache, chin and belly!

I'm so hairy I'll be sprouting hair out of my nostrils and ears next!" We laugh more.

Michael adores Fiona's perfectly carved face, explaining that she has beautifully shaped edges and he often see's people looking her up and down as if she were a super model. I have to agree - her face is sculpted as if hand carved by a perfectionist, and with more confidence she could be quite stunning. But Fiona has been too self-conscious for too long. She started taking the pill when she was thirteen because of the acne, which luckily left no scars, and the doctors suspect this is what has triggered the polycystic ovaries by preventing her body to develop properly at such a young age. It's obviously something she is very upset about. Michael is a very caring man and loved feeling needed and being able to care for Fiona now he could see her insecure side. They became a couple after lent.

"I think Michael is a superior person and the way he looks after kids is amazing," Fiona tells me. "Not that he wears the pants!" she is quick to add.

"If I did, she would only pull them down," Michael laughs.

Fiona had never wanted marriage and although she had been engaged to Anil it had been upon his request rather than her own, which was why it had ended in such heartbreak. During a meal in a restaurant Fiona told Michael that she still believed Anil was the love of her life.

"If Anil walked in here right now," she told him. "I would walk out with him."

Michael knew Fiona too well and nodded. "And I would still be sitting here when you returned."

Nothing Fiona said could turn Michael away and when she saw this she fell further in love with him. Michael organised a surprise picnic on Boars hill, Oxford, by a big tree which had a low branch for Fiona to sit upon while he proposed. He packed blue cheese rolls, hula hoop crisps, a small blanket and rose petals (free from a florist) to be scattered everywhere. He took his guitar and created the perfect set up on a £10 budget that included food and hot chocolate afterwards in a cafe. It was June and it rained constantly. Michael purposefully broke some bread and wine, sang a song, and then coaxed her to sit in the tree – not an easy feat! He looked up at her, satisfied that the tree was the perfect height.

"Fiona, you are the most beautiful woman ever and I love you to bits, will you marry me?"

Michael got his first proper kiss from Fiona. There was another surprise in store for Fiona when Michael took her to the pub: her mother and her close friends were there. There was live piano music playing all her father's favourite songs and everyone was smiling and happy –Fiona had never felt so loved and cared for.

"It was lovely," Fiona sighs. "Michael has such a wonderful way of making people feel special and looking after them."

Eight months later they were married on an amazing £1000 budget with 350 guests! They did this with cream teas in the day and chips on the evening. It was a wonderful day, proving that all you need are those you love around you, although the build up to the big day was hard for Fiona. She cried and drank a lot at this time because she so desperately wanted her father there and missed him more than ever. Fiona's mother had won a raffle prize: a two night break in a hotel. This was their honeymoon. The hotel upgraded their room when they realised. Not having sex before their wedding night had been difficult, especially since neither of them were virgins, but it had been important to them both.

I can't help ask, "I'm curious how you could hold back until your wedding night. If I plan to dedicate the rest of my life to one man I'd at least like a test drive – what if he was rubbish in bed?"

"Michael is musical and has good rhythm so I was convinced he'd be pretty good in the shack," Fiona smiles naughtily. "I wasn't disappointed."

I won't repeat how Michael knew Fiona would be good in bed - it shuts me up along that line of questioning!

They chose not to face IVF, for both financial reasons (they are too young to qualify for a free round of IVF and simply cannot afford it themselves) and what it does to you physically and emotionally. Fiona feels that there is too much pressure on people to go the IVF route if natural conception fails and she doesn't want to have their lives preoccupied with trying relentlessly and technically to conceive. They chose not to adopt because they want to do peace work in the Middle East, and feel it would be unfair to take an adopted child to a foreign country. Fostering seems the obvious route and they can also work with and help the parents too. They currently have three children and are incredibly busy. There is a part of them that hopes, perhaps, one day they might get pregnant naturally but they will not try and will not become preoccupied with it: what will be will be. They get a lot of pressure from those around them, a story I am hearing frequently, being pushed as to when they are having children.

"We've always had it," Michael shrugs. "*When are you guys getting engaged; When are you getting married; When are you having children; Don't take too long, what about seeing our grandchildren?* We just push the pressure away and try not to let it bother us: people don't like minding their own business."

"Life just happens," Fiona says. "And it isn't sweet, easy or predictable."

Chapter 12 - Unfettered Life As A Single Mum

I had been thinking about not being able to have any more children. When the twins were five months old James and I agreed that we wouldn't cope until the twins were older and decided to try for another one, without IVF, when the twins started pre-school. Meeting someone else and having children with a second man was not something I was willing to consider. I had seen others juggling the weekend visits between two difficult ex's and I did not want to be in that position. It would also mean having children in my forties and a bigger age gap. I didn't want to take more time off and be stuck at home again: it was going to be hard enough establishing a new career as it was. As far as I was concerned, this was my time to have children and then I was done.

Finding a new relationship was going to be incredibly hard because I was house-bound, had trust issues and was no longer looking just for me. It was complicated now and my young twins were likely to deter many men. There would be double fathers, mothers, children, grandparents and difficult ex's all around – it sickened me. A lot of mature men had had children, may have had a vasectomy, and didn't want any more. I didn't want to feel bitter or hateful towards James for taking that second pregnancy away from me. If I decided to find a man to have more children with then I could not enter that relationship with an open heart, would have an ulterior motive, and once more enter a life of having sex just to get pregnant. I didn't want the passion killed right at the start.

A local friend, one of the few who still spoke to me at toddler groups, knew and understood how much I had wanted another baby since the twins arrived. She had three children and knew what it was like to want more than one or two children. She didn't judge me negatively but accepted my desire. She told me of a friend she had who asked a guy to get her pregnant – no strings attached – so that she could have a baby and promised not to ask him for anything. He obliged but I didn't think that suited me: I didn't want to know the man. I faced none of these issues with an anonymous sperm donor and she suggested that I did a pro and con list. I had only one con: how would I explain to my child that daddy was coming to pick the twins up but they didn't have a daddy coming for them?

"What about your name?" she asks. "Are you keeping it? That might be an awkward thing, having one child with a different name."

"Well, that's what puts me off having kids with someone else later on. I don't want the twins to be at school with a different name from me, it just gets complicated and shouts "hello, he left me!" so I am keeping the name. That way, any new baby would have the same last name too; schools and strangers would just assume we are all one. I've already tasted people's overly-harsh judgement."

I resented having to keep my married name – it was no longer me – and the thought of having children with a different name was just as offensive to me and felt wrong. I couldn't find a reason not to go ahead. My sister thought I was crazy but had promised to help me in those early weeks. However, she was about to become a grandmother, despite being only four years older than me: I was having children alongside my twenty-year-old niece.

"Ask that gay friend of yours to be your donor," my niece suggests with an innocence I adore and would like to have again.

"Honey, I have fallen out with a long standing friend recently just because I brought a man back to the house, can you imagine how judgemental of any future decisions a friend would become if they had a vested interest in one of my children?"

"Oh yeah, he would interfere all the time."

"Anyone would, they wouldn't be able to help themselves. I want no comeback and no man interfering in my life. I do not want to be dealing with two daddies showing up at weekends and juggling who has who and when."

"What if you have twins?" she laughs.

"Oh, I know, I've thought about that and it could happen. I just have to hope it doesn't."

"Or triplets," she giggles.

Perhaps if I were twenty years younger I would giggle more too. "Or a disabled child or I might get sick, I know. That is why I asked you and your mum to be here in the early weeks if I go ahead with this. With you guys I shall have more help and support than I did when I was married." They didn't like James so didn't visit while I was married to him – he was rude to them – he was rude to everyone. I refused to see it and was told awful stories of how friends had been treated once we had split. With time I received firsthand experience of what it was like when James could not be bothered with you – it was not argumentative but a rude and unpleasant treatment.

At the end of the day, I wanted to focus on my children, career and building a new social network. Men needed more time than I had. Time invested in a new relationship took away time from the children. I was statistically more likely to have a second failed marriage and splitting up was so much harder and emotional when children were involved. Breaking up with a partner was bad enough before but when you still loved someone, and had their children, and had to see them weekly, it was terrible. It was common for women with twins to crave having just one baby. I never experienced a "baby moon" and felt as if I missed out on a magical moment. It was relentless work and panic. I'd been very clear for over twenty years about what I wanted and that hadn't changed. The only thing that had changed was how I did it. I had boy and girl hand-me-downs and the baby could sleep with me. I was concerned about birthday and Christmas presents from grandparents and daddy, the twins would receive them but not a third child, and that would be sad. What if the baby felt jealous of the twins? Was this selfish or not? I was so angry and upset that he had left me and I had not completed my family.

My GP referred me to the hospital for donor insemination as a single mother and, of course, it was going to cost a lot of money. Any money I made from breeding Fudge should be put aside for emergencies. I wouldn't consider IVF at all, even though the consultant told me this was the best way forward. First of all, I needed to be healthy and there for the twins and all the appointments and risks were not fair on them. IVF was not an option. IUI (intrauterine insemination), even without the drugs, was a lot of money I would rather spend on the twins. I discussed this during my CBT course and expected the nurse to be negative or advise against it but she completely understood and explained that she was not there to tell me what to do.

"It sounds to me like you have thought this through thoroughly and made your mind up," she says.

I had. I nod.

"You certainly seem confident about it, which is good; a lot of women are doing this nowadays."

"You don't think it's a bad thing to do?"

"No, not at all. I believe we are all destined to have a certain number of children and if you wanted a big family then that is your heart's desire. If you really want another baby then you really want another baby – that is all there is to it – there's no on/off switch."

"A lot of people think I should be content because I have two already, especially one of each."

"Let them think that. What matters is how you feel."

"Do they think I'm stupid or immature or something? It seems that way."

"I think the problem is that people don't understand big families nowadays. Most people only have one or two children. I bet the friends who voiced concern only have one child, if any?"

I nod – she was good – and it was true. Every friend I had struggled with had a single child, was unable to relate to me with two children let alone specific issues with twins. Probably all they saw was that I had a two for one deal and should be grateful.

"They don't understand and think differently, that is all. Accept it. Accept people's views and opinions for what they are and be true to yourself. You are very confident in ways most women are not and it will be hard for you to find females who relate to or agree with you. Accept it. You like being different and that is how you are. Now, I want to address this feeling of being worthless you have had since you were eleven and how you think you are, at best, average. We did a lot of work on that and your homework looks very positive. I think we've overcome this one now, don't you?"

As with most things, once you started looking into them a whole new world opened up to you. I was told that the waiting list at the hospital was over a year, at the very best, for sperm donation and the nurse who helped me donate my eggs recommends some places to go and find a sperm donor myself. I sometimes found myself thinking about the son I helped to create – were his parents still together? I was not proud of the sort of parents James and I had become, which was ironic since I was worried about my donated son's upbringing. I was not so righteous now. Finding donors was a world unto itself. Married couples, gay couples, single career women, abandoned women like me not wanting the man involved – it was a busy world of activity and my eyes were opened. I was not mad then - it was happening a lot – I was just more open about it than most. I was initially very focused on AI (artificial insemination). I could get a home kit or just simply use a syringe – that seems to be popular and successful – I found it very interesting. I found it amazing that so many couples struggled for years and on the other hand a donor could hand over a pot of sperm and a woman could use a syringe and get pregnant that easily – it was ironic. I found Mr. M, who was very polite and respectful, unlike some who were dangerously and irresponsibly just trying to get unprotected sex. I loved being able to be so open and honest about what I wanted. We arranged to meet up on a night James was having the children but James cancelled on the afternoon – he wasn't feeling well.

"This first meeting is the nerve racking one," Mr. M tells me, incorrectly assuming my bottle had gone. "Always best to get it out of the way."

I loved the easy manner and open way in which he talked. I clicked with him over the phone easily – always a good sign for me. I hesitated, feeling angry at my lack of freedom to go anywhere or do anything, weighing up the risk and the situation. I couldn't afford or even find a babysitter – what should I do? James paid the crèche direct in vouchers, prior to being taxed, and I had to remain on site. Mr. M offered to come over, despite not having met before, and said he understood if I said no. I decide to take the risk, hearing my friends words in the back of my mind, but this would not happen otherwise. I was very nervous as I got dressed and tried desperately to double-fold my stomach, or muffin-top as my niece describes it, into my jeans, even though this was just a discussion about AI.

I caught my breath as I opened the door to a rather tall blonde and muscular man with a gorgeous smile. He was really hot. We had a cup of tea and he told me all about himself, what motivated him, how he had done AI for a number of couples, had nine children from his donations while a student and five since he had been doing it privately. I could see he was very similar to me – open, honest and good-hearted. We clicked and before we knew it two hours had passed. He had a briefcase with all his STD checks and was very professional and sensitive to how awkward I was.

"When are you next fertile?" he sounded like a consultant at the fertility hospital.

"Today is day eleven so now and next week really. I was planning on starting next month if that's OK with you?" we look long and hard at each other.

"Now? Well, I have done NI—"

"NI?"

"Natural insemination. I've done it once before and I have to say you are the most attractive woman I have met in a while, I'd be happy to save you the money and go for NI. It's only an offer, I can't just do it with anyone, and you aren't going to offend me if you still prefer AI, here or at the hospital, I understand it's unusual circumstances. I'm here and I'm flexible in your case."

Despite how it may sound it was delivered in a surprisingly non-cheesy fashion. I had a throat-full of cotton wool and started to shake with nerves. I felt like a teenage virgin. I think it was how muscle-bound he was and his immense height - he was tasty – I was dribbling and trying to hide it. It went against everything I believed in but I wanted him and had no reason not to have a bit of fun while it was on offer. A year earlier I would never have imagined I could even consider something like this but now my whole life and outlook was different. It was insane. However, there was a very attractive man offering himself on a plate and I was very lonely.

"OK," I squeaked.

I was very nervous and there was a brief moment of awkwardness as we went into my bedroom but he was such a gentleman, very reassuring and kind that I was at ease as soon as he kissed me. He was a good kisser, as sensual as I was - we click. Part of me can quite happily take a year getting pregnant with him while another part hoped it was first time because he could be dangerous – I could certainly fall for him. I had not felt this good in a very long time and was glad I hadn't removed the stair gate from the twins bedroom yet. He was obviously very attracted to me too and equally surprised by how well we got on. There was absolutely no awkwardness. It felt right and that surprised me even more. He proudly showed me pictures he had been sent of the children he had helped create. It must be a cracking position for him to be in. It was obviously not about the sex for him, since he mostly donated via AI. He believed in helping all sorts of people have children; gay, married or single. I really respect that. Some people may think I was vulnerable, and in many ways I was, but I was also world-travelled, far from naive and gagging for a sex life. He was genuine and open and lovely to spend time with. Not as closed-minded as so many people I met.

Chores weren't so miserable now that I did them with a mind full of naughty thoughts and a dance in my step. I was much more productive. I was not ignorant to the irony that I now had a man who was very excited about having sex to get me pregnant. He loved it and managed to make me feel special – for the first time in years. I was amazed at how considerate he was towards my feelings, considering he didn't know or care about me, when my own husband had never seemed to care how I felt. They say the best things in life are free and they definitely are. He was taking a HUGE risk doing this with lots of possible CSA cases on his back but he was obviously a very generous man and believed in what he was doing. He was gorgeous, sexy and available – all I was thinking was, "Please do it again, hurry back and do that again!" Some men have it, others make you feel cheap like my fling.

This was much better than going to a clinic; I was successful in business and self-employed from an early age because I was not scared to take risks. I was also very good at judging people's true colours and my father was a middle weight boxer who was gutted at only having girls so taught us all to pack a punch better than any man. I went on to do kick-boxing and could handle myself well. Not many men could put me down physically. I could get the vast majority of men out of my house with minimum hassle if the need be. So the risk was not as great for me as it might be for others. Some friends, the new ones I had made, thought it was wonderful and loved my wild side whereas others, mostly the older friends, were appalled. People assumed the worst or simply liked to gossip any chance they got and relished in putting others down. I wondered if it was because the older friends knew James and I as a couple for so long and were struggling with how fast we had broken up and what I was choosing to do. They hadn't come to terms with it but I had.

I wanted Chris and Beth to have a sibling, it would be good for them, and I had a broody and bitterness issue. I had the best sex I'd had in years and he made me feel better than my husband ever did – this was an eye opener and I was shocked at how much I tolerated as a married woman and how poor my sex life had been. Had I really never had a good lover – ever? It made me realise how good something like this would actually be with someone I loved. There was no going back. I was contented and happy and able to direct my own life and desires – it was empowering. I only hoped I did not get pregnant quickly because it would break James's pride that bit more if I got pregnant easily. I told James what I was doing and he said he understood and didn't mind. I was shocked when he told me that he would consider the children as a package and take all three out together. His response unsettled me and I wondered if he was in shock and didn't understand what was happening to us or if he simply didn't care.

Fudge played me up during her last week of pregnancy, milking the situation for extra attention, showing signs of imminent whelping. I'd been sleeping on a blow up air bed on the floor next to her whelping box. A week of little sleep and the pups hadn't even arrived. This was going to be really hard work – what was I thinking? Now I'd have even less time for the children. I felt selfish and ashamed. One night I awoke to a strange squeaking noise and soon realise a pup has arrived – right on my neck! I sat up carefully and assessed the situation; my hair and ear was covered in a bloody-gloop. Tenderly, I talked to Fudge as I placed the little pup in the whelping pen, a little girl who I later name Honey, and encourage Fudge to follow. The second pup slipped out of its sack as it was born, which I assumed happened with the first one too, and I handed it to mum. Fudge pushed ten puppies out within six and a half hours. The last two were over two hours apart making the entire whelping time close to twelve hours. She bites some umbilical cords down to nothing and they lost copious amounts of blood as I rapidly tried to bandage their slippery jelly-like bodies and apply pressure to stop the bleeding. One pup bled a lot for over half an hour and I almost lost him. As soon as the last one popped out I raced upstairs and had a much needed shower to get the gunk out of my hair. I had expected six to eight puppies for her first litter. Twelve puppies: a surprisingly large first litter. I was immediately worried about her coping: this was a lot of puppies to deal with and she was obviously exhausted. Nine bitches, three dogs – this was great news since bitches were easier to home.

I was up on the hour every hour letting Fudge out with her upset stomach after eating twelve placentas and watching her shit black liquid at all hours - I didn't sleep for more than an hour at a time for the first four nights – similar to when the twins were born. I had to constantly move the puppies back to her before they got cold and died. It was a lot of pressure. I had to monitor bullies too and ensure the weaker ones got fair time on the nipple - this was really hard - nine nipples and twelve puppies. As soon as I got a weak one on the teat another big one pushed her away. This was the part I found the hardest to manage - just as I got them settled Fudge's diarrhea came back and she rushed outside – the fight for milk started all over again upon her exhausted return. She tried to roll on them, crush them, and reduce her workload. I wouldn't let her. I saved them and cuddled her – poor girl - and I thought twins were hard work!

My au pair had the children at a friend's house during the whelping and was a godsend. The first night Fudge pushed a little boy aside and I knew something was wrong with him. So does she. She would not waste time on him when she had so many to look after. I held him, trying to get him warm but he can barely breathe and was slipping away – puppy fading syndrome. It was rare for an entire litter to survive but anything less than a hundred percent was a failure to me. It was a bad attitude to have and I resigned myself to comforting him during his last breaths and cried when he passed away. I wanted to bury him but I was unsure where or how I would have the time. Fudge would smell him in the garden and dig him up and there was no time to go anywhere and bury him and risk the lives of the rest of the puppies. I turned an empty tissue box into a pretty and safe coffin and place him in the black bin. It broke my heart to do so but there were eleven puppies, Fudge and the twins to prioritise. The twins were great: they stayed away with the au pair for a few days and I ran between them and Fudge, recording everything and showing it to them on the camcorder. They loved it and I sneaked them in for a peek when Fudge took a toilet break – it was all very exciting to them and they told everyone at preschool about their puppies.

After a week, Fudge has recovered and was now able to take on the workload alone. I waved goodbye to the au pair sooner than I liked because Fudge had a long pregnancy so I only had help for the first week and had no chance to catch up on sleep. She was a good doting mother and I was overwhelmed with pride. Visits didn't end once they paid a deposit for the puppy – they returned weekly in order to bond with the puppy and brought the entire family each time. Eleven puppies – that was a lot of visitors.

It was madness but the twins loved meeting all the children coming and going from our house and spent hours playing in the puppy pen. The mornings were the worst: I had the twins and all the puppies screaming at me for breakfast as soon as I got up and my back was terrible – I could barely move with the pain. I threw a bowl of cereal at the children and a glass of milk, put the puppies in a different pen with their mash and frantically cleaned out their filthy pen before they finished breakfast. My back made it painful and difficult, especially lifting the puppies in and out. The day was not so bad because I picked up the poo as it happened but overnight they were left alone as I slept so it was positively vile first thing. I ended up with poo in my nails, on my clothes and struggled to stay sane.

I can't remember when I last ate – three days ago? I was bombarded with enquiries because there was a huge demand for fox red puppies at the time; and I seemed to have the only fox red litter. Honey was the first one chosen. I was gutted but relieved: now that she had a home I knew I wouldn't keep one. This woman had pick of the litter, took my first love and first born, I was safe! I planned to keep a puppy from the second litter.

Worming was hilarious: I had to get a thick white liquid paste down all the puppies' throats for three consecutive days. I weighed them, trimmed their nails as they wriggled, checked the little woollen collars I'd made weren't too tight and replaced them with bigger ones if they were and prepared the syringe. They soon cotton on that the worming solution is vile and were remarkably innovative in ways to avoid, cough it up, or spit it out. By the end of each worming I looked like a tribal woman covered in white paint. The twins were having a lot of fun and helped me look after them. I was pleased it was educational and felt less selfish about breeding Fudge. It was actually lovely having a house full of puppies.

Honey's new owners messed me around with the deposit, eventually saying they had changed their mind. It was annoying because they took over a week to do this and I'd turned many people down since all the puppies had gone. It was very hard to get someone to come and view the last puppy – everyone assumed she was a runt. It was a lesson well learned. I began to doubt my decision to have another baby.

The puppies would be gone within two months but the baby would be hard work for a lot longer and I doubted my sister would be as supportive as she claimed – I hardly heard from her now that she had a new boyfriend. I couldn't do it alone. Reality set in and I decided to stop seeing the sperm donor. I would miss his company, the open discussions and how sexy he made me feel. It was the end of an era and I had to come to terms with the fact that the twins and one pregnancy was my lot in life. I was happy with that, I knew how lucky I was and to try for more, given the circumstances, would be selfish and too risky. I was not going back to pregnancy and motherhood in my forties, this was my time, and I happily accept Honey as compensation. She was staying with us.

Progressively, the amount of puppies reduce: four poop's a day less, eight poop's less...was all I thought despite choking up as each one went – the first collected was the most emotional. I had met a lot of lovely people through these puppies and it had been a fantastic experience. I was left with Honey and Fudge. I could afford a nice Christmas with the children and had the reassurance that if anything like the car or boiler had problems I could cover it. My stress levels reduced.

The twins play nicely together, allowing me to do more things than a mother with one or separate aged siblings could. They had a lovely friendship and bond and it was adorable to watch. I remembered how guilty I felt with them as babies, having to settle for half of my time and attention as I poorly juggled them and was relieved to see the precious bond they had as a result of being twins - that guilt had now vanished.

Jude informed me of a writers retreat, an Arvon course, and said I should look into it. I did and there happened to be a cancellation on the November week and they even said I could have a grant to cover half of the cost.

"I'm gutted," I told James, "because I could have done with a week to get my head together but you've only just returned from a holiday in France with your parents and can't take another week off. It would have been nice. There isn't another one until next Summer."

I was astonished when he called me back half an hour later and said, "I've checked with my boss, explained the situation and he agrees that it is a fantastic opportunity. He's letting me have the week off. Go – you deserve it."

It was a last minute dash and I was excited. I wanted to get away. I had taken enough of this hard life. My hands were so dry they were cracked and bleeding. I had no consideration for the twins or how they would take it – I was physically and emotionally drained. Our divorce NISI had just come through. I explained to the twins that I was going away to school for a little while. They stood on the platform and cried hysterically as the train pulled away. Their little faces haunted me the entire journey as I uncontrollably sobbed in front of everyone – the train was full. Even James's eyes welled up. I felt overcome with selfishness.

I spent the first night in a B&B in Shropshire in a converted hay loft. The owner collected me from Craven Arms train station and they were the friendliest of people. I felt as if I had entered normality again. I coloured my hair, shaved my gorilla-like hairy body, applied a face mask, and did some reading and writing before going to bed. I slept for fifteen hours, awaking somewhat more refreshed. I put the kettle on and took a breath of fresh air outside. I was surprised by the amount of sheep immediately in front of me; I wasn't expecting to see them so close. Water was running somewhere; horses neighed; ducks and geese quacked as they played in the river; the dogs were barking. This was the first peace I had known in over two years. The kids should be at preschool now: I'd booked them in for three days this week so he should cope. I bet he just breezes through the week and makes it look incredibly easy. Please God, let me see blood-shot eyes and misery on his face when I return—

I was surprised at how long the day seemed and I was not sure what to do with myself. I dragged out breakfast – a fabulously large fry-up with the most delicious homemade marmalade. I had a cry, a nap, did a very long yoga session overlooking the hills, stepped outside and tipped my head to the sky as I drank in the soft country rain, delicious! It was a good job I stayed in this B&B before my course started because it had given me the chance to unwind and prepare myself emotionally.

I had to check in by four. I immediately came down with the most chronic cough and cold and disrupted the classes and spread my germs – everyone was coughing by the end of it. I felt terrible and should be in bed recovering but I didn't want to miss out on anything – the course was amazing. Initially, I didn't miss the twins at all and conclude that I was a bad mother. If I didn't go back they would always want me, miss me, as they currently did their father instead of my ogre-like exhausted behaviour while coping on my own. They would end up hating me and loving him. Such were my thoughts and emotions but as the week passed and I relaxed I knew that I could never live without them or leave them again. It was a good thing to learn.

The week had changed my life in many ways. I had learned a lot about writing and met a number of wonderful passionate women. Speaking with them and listening in on their conversations made me realise how hard my life was compared to theirs and how far from relaxed I was. I was running at a different pace to everyone here, my mind was bogged down with trouble, life was overcoming me. The cough kept me awake each night, along with the poor journalist sharing my room, and to make me look even worse I was the only smoker standing out in the cold getting my fix. I looked a wreck and I drank too much – what must they think of me! They all seemed so normal and nice – I felt so ashamed of myself for being such an emotional wreck. However, to have a week to step away made it all so clear. I took a deep breath and prepared for change: I knew what I had to do now. On the train journey home I was choking up at the thought of seeing the children again. As I held them in my arms, tears streamed down my cheeks and I realised that I was incomplete without them.

James had done every single task on the list and was red-eyed, unshaven and resembling a tramp. It made me happy. The house was clean and everything was in order – he had done a lot and, most importantly, he had coped and the twins had had a nice week. It felt good to have them back in my arms. James was shocked by how hard each day was and promised to come round two evenings a week and bath the children and put them to bed for me. I was grateful for the help and it was good for the twins to see him. It took a couple of weeks of reminding him of this promise before he grudgingly kept to it. It was helpful, allowed me to finish chores earlier each evening and tolerating his nastiness was worth it.

Chapter 13 – Cliff and Jane

Cliff and Jane strike me as a very practical couple. Their careers as an IT consultant and a nurse is perhaps why and Jane has a clear understanding of fertility problems. They met at University; Cliff was just completing his degree and Jane was doing a conversion course. They bumped into each other, for the first time, at the dive club. For six months they were good friends and spent a fair amount of time together. Many student friends thought they were secretly dating, but they were not, until Jane became impatient with the relationship and began to question their friendship. One night, after far too much alcohol, she confronted Cliff about it. In fact, she was so confrontational, they laugh, that she almost pushed Cliff over the balcony they were standing on.

"So, are we going out or not?" She demanded.

Cliff, looking over his shoulder at the impending drop below, unable to take another step backwards, was forced to answer.

"Yes, we are," he replied, almost desperately.

They kissed and it was all decided right there and then. They enjoyed student life and, three years after they met, moved in together. They shared a flat before deciding it was financially better to buy a house. At this point, they had been together for six years. Jane progressively became stressed and unhappy. She assumed it was the stress from her nursing job and was given counselling to help. She was also suffering from chronic migraines. As it turned out, she was desperately broody and wanted a baby and was blatantly aware that Cliff did not. Her friends told her that she was mad staying with a man who didn't want children, when she so obviously did, and advised her against it. They weren't married and both had separate goals. However, Cliff wasn't as set against having children as Jane assumed, he just wasn't particularly bothered either way. With her friend's encouragement, Jane stopped hiding her broodiness, faced it and opened up to Cliff. He surprised her with his compassion and understanding. There was no arguing, no long discussion, it was simple.

"I really want a baby," she sighed.

"Well, we should get married then," he smiled.

They married within three months at a small registry office and went to a pub for lunch afterwards. They booked a table at the pub, for a small group of them, and when the pub realised that it was actually for a wedding party they were furious because they would have charged more – exactly why the practical couple didn't tell them and just booked as normal. It was only their closest family and uneventful since the main purpose was to satisfy Cliff's strong belief that marriage was essential when it came to having children. Jane was more than happy. Cliff had resented years of peer pressure from those around them, the typical irritating questions like, "when are you getting married?" and "Are you trying for children?" They had, as a couple, received many hurtful comments, especially from parents and put it down to that generation and how they thought. Cliff's parents said things that were particularly difficult to swallow but Jane's parents seemed to show more understanding.

"I just wanted Jane to be happy," Cliff said. "I was more laid back about what would happen."

They began trying for a baby, which grew increasingly difficult with Cliff working away Monday to Friday and the long and flexible shifts of a nurse. At times, she would travel to visit him and their sex life soon became very functional.

"It just lost its spunk," Jane says.

"It was horrible repeatedly doing it for a purpose," Cliff agrees.

It didn't help that Jane had problems with coming off the pill, which she had been on for a very long time because of her problematic periods. Due to this, the GP was closely monitoring her and there was already suspicion that at thirty-four, and Cliff a couple of years older, they might have problems conceiving. Jane wonders if she had an early miscarriage, one year after trying to conceive, when she experienced a very large period which lasted a lot longer than previous ones. However, with her periods being as heavy and irregular as they were it was hard to tell. A pregnancy test, shortly after she began to bleed, showed positive, but a scan three days later showed no life at all. She bled for four weeks.

    The GP referred her earlier than normal, due to her periods, and since they were already on the system and uncertain whether or not she had been pregnant naturally, they decided to carry on with the referral. With the help of a few little white lies, since all hospital rules differ, they got treatment earlier than normal: time was against them and her nursing background let Jane know, in no uncertain terms, what lay ahead. The staff merely wanted to push them straight down the IVF route without doing any proper tests on Jane: she will never get over how poor her treatment was. The tests they received were limited and pointless but they followed the consultants request to put them straight through for IVF, assuming they would probably end up there regardless, and there was no point in alienating the consultants who would be treating them. Then, it happened quickly. Cliff's sperm was sluggish, which is not unexpected since sperm fluctuates, and the delay in doing the test, as it got "mislaid" didn't help. His second sample was borderline and his sperm's mobility was less than it could be. Cliff immediately knew that this was down to his lifestyle: working away, living in hotels and restaurants and having a drink with most meals. They knew that if he changed his lifestyle, which he did, and tried naturally for longer, they might get pregnant normally. However, since the hospital had done no proper testing on Jane, they had no idea if there was a problem on her side. As recommended by their consultant, conscious of their age and with the technology right there waiting for them, they signed up for their one and only round of NHS IVF treatment. Jane had set her mind on only having one round of IVF and freezing whatever embryos she could, partly for financial reasons and partly because of the stress of the whole experience. At first, she didn't realise that Cliff was prepared to pay for more rounds and already had a contingency plan for further funding. Jane knew nothing about what money he had and didn't realise that he could afford it.

"It was incredibly considerate and sweet of him and took the pressure off me," she explains. "I am very cautious with money and didn't want to spend any on IVF when we should use that money for our children. I was determined to only have the NHS funded round of IVF and no more."

They look at each other with a knowing smile.

"But I don't know if I would have continued to feel that way," she added.

"You see desperate people going bankrupt and obsessed with repeated rounds and I didn't want us to go there but I thought we should try two or three," Cliff said.

Jane did acupuncture; something I agree is a powerful aid. Jane is convinced it was a massive contributing factor to their success. Cliff claims he saw the physical difference in Jane and her behaviour following acupuncture.

"She was so much more relaxed and at ease," he nods. "It was obviously benefiting her regardless of anything else. However, I wonder how much of it is the actual acupuncture and how much of it is the advice and counselling the therapist provided during the treatment."

"It's the acupuncture," Jane insists.

"But you don't remember everything that you came back and told me. I remember all the things you used to say and the therapist often put your mind at ease and said the right thing."

Jane ponders upon this for a moment before replying. "You might have a point there - she was fabulous. Mind you, I only did it for a month before IVF, not as long as they recommend, but it was lovely."

When Jane began the drugs, it had little effect upon her personality and she merely shrugged her way through them. She admits it might be because she is a nurse and had a fairly knowledgeable and relaxed approach to it all.

"Except for that one time," Cliff interrupts with a smile.

"Oh, yes, I was getting to that," she laughs. "I had one major wobble when they tested my FSH levels and they were really high - I freaked out and completely lost the plot! I just assumed that I wouldn't be allowed to have IVF now and just lost it, it was all for nothing, all over, and we had gotten nowhere and we had no more money to try again. I went into panic mode."

It was also winter time and her work was putting great pressure upon her, as it often does for nurses at this time of year, and she didn't think to ring and check the situation with the clinics. This is one of the times, she admits, that her knowledge as a nurse made matters worse because she jumped to the worst case scenario. She didn't get time during her shift to call and check and just became increasingly emotional. Until Cliff, all calm and collective during a frantic phone call, assured her that it would be fine – they could just reduce the amount of drugs she was taking. The obvious hadn't occurred to her, she couldn't think clearly, and the panic subsided, she returned to her calm, controlled normal self.

"Cliff, was she really that good on the drugs?" I ask. "I find it hard to believe that she was unchanged, they played such havoc with my emotions."

"Well, that is one of the advantages of being away at work all week," he winks.

"I found the drugs that you sniff the worst, they sent me doolally," I said.

"That's what I was on when I had the wobble," she smiled.

The consultant had described the procedure with the injections and Cliff, apparently, went as white as a sheet when he suggested that sometimes the husband did the injections for their wives. Jane stayed quiet at the time but admits that she had absolutely no intention of letting Cliff near her with a needle. She was, granted, the person trained in such a field.

"It's a shame really, I could have gotten into it," Cliff laughs.

"Yeah right, there was no way you were coming near me!" Jane declares.

"I had a lovely vision of standing in a room and throwing dart-like needles at your bum!"

She rolls her eyes in exasperation. He has joked all the way through this interview and I don't think it is just his way of dealing with things, he is just a generally funny and good natured guy. Jane was more worried about her work and how busy she was: she might forget or miss the drugs the way things were going, it was the usual winter madness you get in hospitals and her chaotic shifts didn't help. They reached the egg-retrieval part and she had twelve viable eggs – a good number – but she grimaces as she explains that nothing prepared her for the vast amount of pain that she went through.

"No woman can expect that. All the training in the world doesn't prepare you for such pain as what you have once those eggs are removed. When your fallopian tubes fill up with water the pain is immense and I have a very high pain threshold. For three days afterwards I was in agony and was frequently close to fainting, which was completely out of character for me," she shakes her head.

She sat on the sofa and only got up to go to the toilet, and only when she absolutely had to. Cliff grew increasingly worried at this point, more concerned that they had damaged her in some way and, by way of some freak accident, caused her to be incapable of ever having children from this day forth - something he knew would break her heart. He had been perfectly fine until the egg-retrieval but now he was consumed with worry. I asked about his part in producing the sample and he shook his head and cringed.

"It was just too clinical and weird. I mean, my wife is having a major operation in one room and I am expected to go into another room and feel all saucy?" he sighed. "I couldn't do it. They weren't happy but because I lived so near I insisted on going home and did it there. At least that way I couldn't hear the lab assistants talking while I did it. There was no way I could have done it in that room under those circumstances. They just grudgingly accepted my instance that I was going home and it was all right there, in the privacy of my own house. I mean, who knows, they might be spying on you in those rooms!" he laughed. "My number one paranoia was that they had some sort of camera in there watching me or something. I mean, come on, my wife is having her eggs harvested as I am supposed to come? Who timed that? What a bizarre way of doing it!"

"I agree," I say. "You think they'd at least wait until it's over for one of you. So you went home? You didn't get the milkman or postman to produce a sample for you then?"

"No way, I am more than capable in my own home."

As far as Cliff was concerned, he was fine the moment he handed over his sample; his part was over and he felt immensely relieved. He almost handed it over to the wrong receptionist at one point, who wasn't paying attention and half-baked went to take it before he realised that something wasn't right about this – just in time! Now it was all out of his hands and the relief was immense. Now, it was just a matter of waiting for the phone call the following morning. Ten had fertilised – fantastic news! But the good news didn't last and the numbers started dropping. Jane was terrified that they would want to put the embryos back in three days later, as she was still in so much pain, but they waited. On day three the number of embryos had reduced to six. The nervousness increased. Day five arrived and there were only two left. Neither was good enough to be frozen and they had both implanted: two low quality embryos from twelve eggs. They waited with bated breath. Cliff was worried that she would miscarry. The day of the pregnancy test arrived. She awoke at five in the morning, managed to wait until seven and, at this time, was certain that she wasn't pregnant. She had been getting pains and cramps and was convinced it was bad news.

"I did the stick and waited with a calm numbness that prevented any emotions from taking over," she tells me, looking sideways at Cliff.

It was positive. She went back to bed, told Cliff and then they both went back to sleep – it was just one more stage they had passed, nothing more, no excitement at this point. I asked if her suspected miscarriage prevented her from being excited about it and she nodded, saying that was a great influencing factor and she didn't allow herself to get excited for a very long time. At each point she expected, or was at least prepared for, the worst. Because they had been very open about the IVF they had to update people on the progress and they found that the hardest part about it. Jane sent a text to everyone "pregnancy test is positive."

"I wouldn't allow myself to say that I was pregnant," she said looking down.

She doesn't remember when she became happy about the pregnancy or allow herself to enjoy it but it was after the twenty week mark. The first scan interested Cliff more for the technology than the images bouncing about on the screen. He found the equipment amazing. Jane was plain nervous and hoped she would just be able to tick another milestone off the list – another stage passed. To her, the result was all that mattered; she showed no enjoyment or excitement about the little bean on the screen. It was her job, she believes, that takes the thrill away. To her, all that mattered was finding out whether it was one or two, and she was relieved to find it was one – knowing all the additional complications that twins can bring to the table. They were having a baby - one more stage achieved. Now, she was focused on the neucal scans, having a disabled child, and so on and so forth. She questioned herself about whether or not she would be able to terminate, after all they had gone through, if that were the case.

"It's all so vague," Cliff explains. "They know nothing and on this basis of knowledge you are supposed to make some major decision about the life of a child and whether or not to terminate. To be honest, it shocked me that we were expected to make such a decision on such wishy-washy information."

They had a neucal scan booked at fourteen weeks, since there were no earlier slots available, but by then she was too big and they couldn't do it. Jane was livid and now faced an anxious wait for all the blood tests to be done later in pregnancy. When the results from the blood tests finally came through it surprised her how hard she found it to open the letter. Her fingers shook and it took her several deep breaths and attempts to get there. It was low risk. Suddenly, she was overwhelmed with the feeling that it was all too good to be true.

"To be honest," she says, "I would have preferred to skip the blood tests but Cliff was insistent upon having them done.

"Nothing, absolutely nothing, prepares you for the pressure of having to make such a decision," Cliff says with conviction and a face that shows the seriousness with which he approached it.

Pregnancy suited Jane and it was a wonderful experience for her. In fact, she felt healthier than she had ever felt, not to mention being a more balanced and "normal" person compared to her usual stressed state. Once more, there was a lack of appointments for the twenty week scan and they scheduled her in late, but Jane put her foot down this time and managed to get in on time. They chose not to find out the sex, and escaped to the Lake District on a much deserved holiday. They climbed mountains that Jane admits she should perhaps have avoided considering her state, but it was somewhere during these hikes that she relaxed and, at last, allowed herself to embrace pregnancy. The worry left her. Finally, she could breathe.

Jane went to a late meeting at work and everything seemed fine. She went to bed with the usual kicking and discomfort in her ribs. During the night she awoke with the need to open her bowels, as had often happened during the week, but when she got back into bed the same feeling came over her again. It felt odd this time and she knew something was up. She rang Cliff and then the hospital. The hospital wanted Jane to wait for Cliff to return home so he could take her to a consultancy led unit because she was only thirty-six weeks pregnant. Jane became a little worried that her contractions were too fast and even thought her waters had broken. She went to have a bath and think about what she should do but as she undressed she noticed some blood. Her nursing training kicked in and she knew she needed help: she called an ambulance.

She had increasingly painful contractions and it took her three attempts just to get down the stairs. The paramedics arrived, saw she was close and took her into the lounge shouting out orders at each other to get towels, hot water and more heating. All this had taken less than an hour from her first bowel movement. Meanwhile, Cliff received a phone call from one of the paramedics at 01:30, while working away, so he hurriedly checked out of the hotel and raced home. Jane overheard the paramedics talking about her and how they don't want her to give birth in the ambulance but a different hospital was concerned that she was only thirty-six weeks and wanted her in. The paramedics told her to stop pushing and rushed her into the ambulance. Upon arrival at the hospital she was eight centimetres dilated. From the start of labour to full dilation was a mere five hours. She was ready - and surprisingly calm. There was no time for pain relief except for gas and air since it had all happened so fast and after forty minutes of pushing, the baby was stuck.

Cliff arrived at the house to witness what looked like a disaster zone: mess and blood everywhere in the lounge and no Jane! He raced to the hospital, unsure of which one they had taken her to and had to Google which hospital she had abbreviated on her rushed note. He got there just in time. Since the baby was stuck, they wanted her to sign a form approving a spinal, which she was in too much pain and discomfort to be able to sign, so they helped her and proceeded just as Cliff arrived. The spinal was horrendous but brought on instant relief to the excruciating pain. While it was happening, her training told her of all the dangers and risks of paralysis if she moved during the procedure but her contractions made it difficult to remain still. She was terrified. Somehow, and Jane cannot believe how she managed it, she remained still long enough for the spinal to be done, and Cliff ended up covered in bruises from where she held onto him during the painful contractions to ensure she didn't move. He took it well. It was like a six inch nail going into her back, Jane describes, obviously disliking the memories of it all. The pain relief made it all worthwhile.

The spinal was in preparation of a caesarean, since the baby was back-to-back, but they managed to get her out with forceps. Josie was born weighing 5lb10oz and perfectly healthy considering how early she was. Cliff, not much for details when it comes to the birth of his daughter, was more fascinated by the Morgan Freeman look-a-like obstetrician.

"It was like I was in that film, Bruce Almighty, and this obstetrician was playing God with the birth of baby Josie - it was Morgan Freeman's big moment bringing her into the world," he laughs. "It was surreal and very odd. I can't get that man out of my head!"

They offered Josie to Cliff to hold but he turned his nose up at how messy she was. "Can you do that shake "n" vac thing first please, she's too yucky," he joked.

A clean little Josie was then presented to him and he got to hold his little girl. Neither of them seemed too moved or concerned by the whole birthing experience. Jane was perhaps in a little shock, not really believing that Josie was truly her baby for the first day or so but that soon changed. They had to bottle-feed her 20ml of formula, with frequent urgency, so there was no time to try to establish breastfeeding. Every time Jane tried to master it, Josie failed to suckle and the nurses were far too busy to provide help. Jane spent her time expressing and bringing on her milk supply. She was moved into a cubicle with Josie and that old feeling that it was all too good to be true came back to haunt her. Then, to her horror, Josie went blue.

Jane panicked on the inside and froze on the outside. She didn't know what to do. It lasted merely seconds and Josie returned to her normal colour once more but alarm bells were ringing and Jane knew something wasn't right. Her training as a nurse was more of a hindrance than a help because only the worst case scenarios popped into her mind and drove her crazy with worry. Cliff arrived and Jane was too worried about the baby to notice how white and sick he looked: he had just overheard a story that a mother had recently died of post-natal eclampsia merely nine days after giving birth. He was sick with worry about all the things that could go wrong.

When Jane told him about Josie turning blue he almost vomited. He grabbed a nurse who looked at Josie, who now looked fine, and Jane grew increasingly concerned that they would think she was a silly new mum over-worrying but Josie turned blue again and the nurse was there to witness it. Josie had some time in SCBU, the special care baby unit, for monitoring. She had very bad reflux and was sorted out quickly enough with special formula. After a week in hospital, breastfeeding was finally established. The reflux stopped Josie from sleeping during the day and she would only sleep on Jane, who was very tired, at night.

Cliff has absolutely no regrets about having the child he didn't particularly crave. In fact, he bonded with her instantly, not for any particular reason he remembers, but she was his darling little girl immediately. It was Jane who took a couple of days to accept that Josie was hers and bond with her and she has since embraced every moment of motherhood with gusto.

"I so desperately wanted to be a mother and have loved every single stage of it all," she sighs happily. "Don't get me wrong: I wouldn't have liked each stage to have lasted any longer than it did. I don't understand why people don't want to breastfeed, it is for such a short time in your life, and it has been such a wonderful experience, well, after the first three months of difficulty getting into it."

With the reflux sorted out it is the nights that become hard because Josie finds it hard to settle and wakes Jane constantly. They have great parents who offer tremendous support by staying every couple of weeks and doting on Josie, allowing Jane to get some much needed sleep and recover. I ask about their sex life and whether they have reclaimed it yet. Awkward smiles and lack of eye contact follow as they confess it is far from normal or anything like it was and Jane is particularly worried about it.

"I am petrified that he might go off with someone else," she says, as Cliff takes hold of her hand lovingly. "I know you and one other friend who have had their husbands walk out on them so early on and knowing how easily that can happen terrifies me. You and my friend didn't see it coming, you have both told me how shocked you were, so I'm profoundly concerned about the same happening to me."

However, having a baby, now almost a year old, is exactly as they both imagined it to be and it is a welcome change to their lives.

"Our relationship had been stagnant for a while," Jane tells me. "We were doing the same old things that had become boring: clubbing, eating out, socialising - something was missing and everything else felt empty. This was exactly what we needed. I love it!"

"It's challenging and exhausting, more so for Jane, but life is one hundred percent better," Cliff adds.

They are both beaming with joy and holding hands like young lovers.

Chapter 14 - Exultation For A Fresh Start

I enjoyed being a single mum more than I expected. I still felt lonely sometimes but it was not as lonely as when I was with James. Brief conversations at playgroups and school runs suffice and having two doting Labradors follow me everywhere was marvellous. I suppose I was one of those odd characters who preferred dogs to people: they're trustworthy, loyal and dependable and they lacked the dark side we humans had. Children and dogs don't play games and I knew where I stood with them.

I had always been a loner, and do not know why I hadn't realised this before. As a young teenager, I preferred day-long hikes and read obsessively, entering an imaginary world without real people. I went into Information Technology, one of the most unsociable fields a woman could select, and spent a large amount of time alone with computers working unsociably long hours. No one had called in a while, despite my desperate emails and texts. If I called them, and they actually answered, I was rushed off the phone – it was never a good time. Most didn't answer and I'd heard lots of women proclaim they wouldn't take phone calls after the kids were in bed as they needed the quiet time with their partner. It left people like me even more stranded.

I would always give my friends all the time in the world when they needed me, even at late hours when I knew they had drank too much and were reaching out; I was there for them. It was especially bad when PMS hit and I went insane. I couldn't believe how pre-menstrual I had become and the darkness was incredible. I knew there was something seriously wrong with me. I started keeping a diary to find a pattern because the GP kept fobbing me off with depression and hormones.

I still had days where I was unable to grasp the fact that he actually walked out on me. Some days I stared into space and wondered how on earth he could have been with me so long and then just left me to handle one year old twins all alone with ill-health. I should never have been put through all this so soon after having them. I felt betrayed and let down. I think I shall always feel disappointed that he was the father to my children. It was hard to forgive. I struggled with the status of a divorced woman and single mum. This wasn't what I wanted. He was text book: he couldn't handle my lack of attention and loathed the hard work of two babies. He preferred a life of peace and whirled in to play super-dad every now and then and looked really cool while grumpy old mother struggles with the long and exhausting days.

It was scary when I heard loud noises outside or the dog barked at night and there was only me to protect the children – there had already been one attempted burglary and the back door was dented – Fudge scared them away. A man appeared at my neighbours with flowers and wine one Thursday evening asking where I lived and caring nothing for my reputation. I knew he was a local married man trying his luck but was not sure which one. It was shocking. Just because my husband left me doesn't mean I lack morals and become an easy shag, despite my fling during my emotional breakdown. Fortunately, my neighbour didn't tell him and I never answer the door at night. I had attracted a number of unhappily married men and I wasn't impressed by it at all.

It reminded me of when I worked in Germany and lay in my hotel bed ignoring the soft knocks, little notes and flowers at my door, always past midnight, always when the married men had drank enough to build up the courage to approach me. I will not be anyone's "bit on the side" – I deserved better than that and I would never steal another woman's man. People had affairs regardless of whether they were married or not and I would not do something I would hate done to me. I was not going to change my principles just because I was lonely. I had no respect for cheaters and cannot sleep with someone I can't respect.

Losing my friends had been harder than losing my husband: I did not see that coming either. Several divorced and widowed women, who have experienced the same, have told me we were seen as a threat and might lure their husbands. Friends want to do "couple" things; their insecurities make them scared that it was something they might catch; they didn't know what to say to you; they didn't want to take sides; they didn't want to be around anyone depressed or experiencing something they were terrified of and their fear made them pretend you didn't exist - the excuses were endless. I'd spoken to divorced, widowed and those diagnosed with cancer – it was the same story - friends often act the same and let you down with their sudden vanishing act. I had built up new friends, since having the twins, to lose them so quickly the minute he left and it was incredibly hard to meet new people given the circumstances. When their children were sick and not allowed into nursery I took them in as a favour so they could still go to work. I had several children one week with chicken pox. We used to meet weekly, as they still do without me, and I was dumped the same week James dumped me. That was no coincidence. I felt used and let down and at high risk of being incredibly bitter and horrible to be around. I seemed to be the only older single woman in the neighbourhood. Writing this book and interviewing couples I knew or had only just met had been my therapy, sanity and companion.

"It's the tone people use when speaking to me," I told one single mum. "It's belittling."

"I know exactly what you mean," she nods. "It's as if you're a bad smell."

"Why? Divorce is common nowadays, not socially embarrassing, so why do they talk down to you as if you're scum or, as you say, a bad smell? I need support right now, people being nice to me, I feel rejected and low enough as it is, so why do they treat me like this?"

"I don't know, it's weird and that's why I set up a single parent's group, we all say the same. It's horrible. If you have any friends that stay with you throughout all this then they become golden friends and you see them in a different light: treasure them – they're rare."

I can think of three but they're still unable to visit. The current single groups are too far away for me and I'd failed to build any interest in a local one. It was the wrong time; there was a local one but all the children were grown up now and their mother's had new relationships.

"I'm fed up with the phone calls or texts out of the blue that start a fight," I moan.

"Yes, I had that. They'll find all sorts of petty reasons to fall out with you and make it your fault – it eases their guilt for dumping you in your time of need. Some use it to cut off for good and others make up with you when everything is OK again."

"I'm either a bad mum making decisions they can't bear to watch me make, which has hardly been devastating, or invite them out too often for their liking and they accuse me of making them feel pressured. I invited one girl to a comedy night and received a vile text stating that she was not going through a divorce and I failed to appreciate that she had a baby and a husband to put first and couldn't go out with me. I thought that was really harsh. I am desperate for company but it's not like I'm able to go out often or organise much."

"I know but that's their guilt and the nasty text messages show that they are angry that you've made them feel guilty when they know you need them. They turn trivial things into major offences to get out of being a supportive friend. It's selfish. I stopped inviting people and decided to let them invite me if they wanted to."

"Well, my counsellor said I should let them know I'm free – that they probably feel awkward asking me – thinking I can't join them. I was invited out constantly in the twins first fourteen months, while I was still married, and it takes nothing to invite someone for an afternoon coffee. I was just trying to be clear like my counsellor advised. Did you get invited out when you stopped asking?"

"No."

It was sad. Neither of us should have to go through such things after our husbands walked out on us – isn't that enough to deal with? Older divorced women faced the same a generation ago, I was reliably informed, and set up a new social circle when they re-married. Times had not changed unless you were in a built up area with many people in your situation. A number of birthday parties the twins were invited to in their first year weren't repeated in their second year. I was upset that they had to suffer – they already came from a broken home so young. They needed to be able to go around to other people's houses to play with other people's children but I hoped time changed that and they were treated equally in the neighbourhood as they got older and established their own friends.

I find it hard not to be bitter when I overhear my old circle of friends talking about the house visits they've had that I wasn't invited to – they lack tact. The play dates, coffee mornings and occasional evening get-togethers continue now without me. I was slowly building up a new network of friends that I could trust, from meagre pickings, and preschool gave them social interaction with other children their age. Old friends were resurfacing but I now had trust issues and preferred my own company. I couldn't be bothered with dating or boyfriends or friends; mostly because I was so busy and tired. I went to bed early and got up to do yoga at five thirty. The irony that the social awkwardness I felt during the years of infertility was now closely mimicked as a divorced mother was not lost on me. I had learned from this and often sent flowers or cards to people for no reason other than they were feeling low – I considered others much more than I used to. I guarded myself against those wanting to take advantage of me while I was vulnerable or kick me while I was down.

Christmas was looming and my emotions were running wild. I was scared of spending it alone. This was not how it was supposed to be after all the years of wanting children. To make matters worse, on 9th December his parents moved into a house down the road from me. I preferred the ninety minute drive between us. I had no idea they were selling their house let alone moving here and was upset: this was my space and my home and I hated feeling as if they were watching me. I dreaded going to the shops in case I bumped into them because I hadn't had chance to do my hair and didn't want to be called a slag again.

I didn't enjoy Christmas. I didn't expect to, being my first without James, and I only hoped to survive it. My sister from up North, her boyfriend, two nieces, one with a new baby, and one teenage nephew came for a few days, didn't lift a finger, trashed the house and offered no money towards the huge cost of food. She was also going through a divorce and he was not giving her any CSA or support so she couldn't afford it but then neither could I. I struggled to cater for everyone and had little time for the twins. I asked them to keep the lounge floor clean but I was ignored and my daughter tripped on a blanket (all the teenagers had to have a massive blanket over their laps on the sofa) and split her forehead open. There was blood everywhere and I was tearful, holding Beth, wondering if she needed stitches.

Twenty minutes later my niece dropped her nephew, the three month old baby, and his mum, my other niece, was in tears too. It was too much drama for me. Beth was OK and I was not leaving my sister and her children to watch the twins any longer while I cooked and cleaned constantly. Even when asked, no one would do a thing and I was expected to wait on them. They wouldn't even take their plates into the kitchen. It annoyed me. The large expensive turkey was in the oven and I didn't care whether we ate or not. I played with the twins and their new toys all afternoon and had a nice time. My sister and her boyfriend eventually figured out that I was not doing anything else so attempted to get the vegetables cooked. We didn't eat until after nine on Christmas evening but at least I'd spent some time playing with my children.

The plan had been to get the vegetables ready on Christmas eve but my sister and her boyfriend got drunk at the pub and refused to come home until after midnight. I refused to do it all myself and went to bed. I was no longer depressed at the thought of spending a Christmas alone. I loved my sister and her children dearly but they were an idle and inconsiderate lot and I was already feeling low enough about my first Christmas without James. I was relieved that I gave up on the idea of having another baby since it was clear I lacked the support I needed and now felt stupid for even considering it. I had nothing to complain about and I had heard so many heartbreaking stories compared to mine. I had a beautiful son and daughter. I had not been thinking rationally.

My mother-in-law's face unexpectedly appeared at my lounge window and dread seeped through my pores as the twins saw her and naturally got all excited. It was barely five weeks since they moved here. I was on edge for the next unscheduled visit and couldn't help but notice every car that slowed down outside my house. I felt completely tormented by her.

From the money I had made from selling the puppies I let the twins give their dad an all inclusive holiday to Egypt in January as his Christmas present. January was always a difficult time for him and his depression and I wanted him to be at his best for the children. After all, when he walked out on me I had ran the visas sky high, purchasing everything I thought the twins might need until I could return to work, without a care in the world how they would be paid off. I had half expected to lose the house at the time and was in panic mode. In the divorce he had agreed to take them all on and refused any money from me towards them. The holiday eased my guilt along with the gratitude that he had given me a week away.

I tried hard to be positive about the parents-in-law living locally – at least James had somewhere to have the twins so I didn't have to be around him as much – he could not or did not want them where he rented; I wondered if he was living with her. When they returned, I would keep them up late with a movie and popcorn and we fell asleep in my bed together. I focused on how lovely it was to have them back and to have the chance to miss them. I heard of exhausted parents with no break and knew I had it good.

His parents offered to do a tip run for me – I gratefully accepted. They explained that it will be a quick stop, they were in a rush, so we agreed that I would close the blinds so that the twins didn't see them and get upset with just a fleeting visit. I was on the toilet upstairs with the twins playing in my bedroom. I never shut the bathroom door since it was only me and the twins. I walked out to find my mother-in-law at the top of the stairs. I screamed – her figure in the dark giving me a sudden fright. Then, as I realised who it was, and the twins saw her and got all excited, I was shaking with anger and embarrassment. I couldn't believe that she had let herself in and came up the stairs. She left within a couple of minutes, just wanted to say hello, she explained, and the twins were crying and screaming because they wanted to see her and didn't understand the fleeting visit. I said nothing and concentrated on settling the twins. I was furious but more than anything I was embarrassed.

I'd learned a lot since my journey with IVF began. From little things, such as realising just how loud my family really was and that Darwin was correct, I directly evolved from the Siamang monkey probably as little as two or three generations ago! Watching the Siamang monkey's shout at each other reminded me of Sunday afternoon's with my parents and I burst out laughing. To bigger things, such as realising how strong I was in many ways yet how weak I was too. I had changed so much as had my outlook on life. I began to see a lot of people stuck in unhappy marriages and felt the relief that I was free and even enjoying being single. It was easier in many ways. I was liberated and knew exactly what sort of a man I should look for in the future when I was ready.

My wedding was half full of people I barely knew, or had never met, who hated me because of the things she had told them. It was a strange wedding in a way; my half of the guests got up and went outside between every course and had a fag or two rapidly crammed in, while his half sat watching hawk-like - it was awkward and strained. I remembered sitting there and watching the two families refusing to interact with each other and wondering where I actually belonged – not with either side. But James and I had each other regardless of where we came from and loved each other deeply. We both considered ourselves the black sheep in our families and were not close to any of them.

My own family were dysfunctional in a different way and all I learned from my parents was how to smother emotions with alcohol. I found it so sad how families could be with each other. The rivalry, jealousy, control and power games all seemed so trivial and pointless. I read that it was common for people to marry into families that mimic their own. I couldn't help but marvel at the power of the mother-in-law and had to admit that I no longer laughed at jokes about it.

Potty training was the worst thing I had ever had to do: my life was literally full of shit. The twins and puppy having accidents at the same time and my having to move faster than the speed of light to empty the potty before the puppy did was the most disgusting thing I had ever experienced. It was tedious and unrewarding work. Chris was easy and within a week of his second birthday he was out of nappies and dry day and night. Beth took a year longer because she didn't want to do what Chris was doing and rebelled stubbornly. I was tremendously glad when it was over.

Walking the twins, a puppy and a dog was no mere feat and despite the occasional moments of fear and panic I managed to make it fun every day. I had the four children I'd always wanted, with the two dogs, and each walk made me feel happy that this was my family. I liked it. I was even getting better on the bike, more difficult to manage with the four of them and the twins beat each other up if they were in the trailer together. Therefore, I put one twin and the changing bag in the trailer and the other twin on a seat behind me. The puppy soon figured out why her mother didn't run in front of the bike. It was a massive effort to get the bike on the car but we all had a lot of fun once we got there.

I tried to become a foster parent but having young twins put everyone off and the only social worker willing to visit me came for an hour, was rude, unpleasant and made me feel nervous and uncomfortable. She had only known me an hour and I had to answer all her questions – therefore talking a lot. She was supposed to wait for her manager to return from holiday to discuss me so I was surprised to receive a standard rejection letter two days later. I asked for a reason and was informed in writing that I talked too much to be considered for fostering. It was the weirdest experience. I was a chatterbox, especially since I was alone and without adult company and often do burst into conversation when an opportunity arises, but I was also a good shoulder to cry on. I knew she had taken an instant dislike to me and left me feeling appalled that these were the sort of people in charge of the children in need in our society. There was no reason I couldn't at least do respite foster care on the weekends the twins were with their father. It seemed so wrong. It was an experience I didn't wish to repeat and made me more sympathetic towards friends of mine who had tried to adopt and had been treated poorly. I had no intention of putting myself through anything like that again and offering to foster in the future. They didn't even take any references.

James finally got the promotion he was after and for about three days he was jubilant. Then, he was down in the dumps again.

"I thought you would be excited about your promotion for a little longer than a few days," I said.

"I know. I've wanted it for so long and now I've got it I just feel a bit lost and it's not all I expected it to be," he sighs.

"You just don't know how to be grateful! Your brother is on round eight of IVF and you have no appreciation how easy you have had everything and still you're miserable because your promotion didn't fix all your life problems!"

I find it frustrating but realise, after I'd said this, that it was typical of depression. He focused on one thing, and if only that one thing happened then the whole world would be better, and when that one thing was achieved it didn't change the feelings inside – I'd watched him do this for years. He continued to refuse to do a thing about it and sulked his way through each week. Someone who had known both James and I suggested he had Asperger's syndrome, something she had a lot of experience with, which would explain his behaviour.

It didn't matter what caused him to do the things he did: boarding school syndrome, another woman, depression, a breakdown, Asperger's or plain selfishness. Perhaps I needed him to have a bigger reason for leaving other than simply not wanting to be with me. I cared not whether a mother was a drug addict, an alcoholic, suddenly unlovable, temporarily fat or just a pain in the neck: it was the man's duty to be there for his children - particularly in the early years - especially with twins. I read stories of the lengths some men went to, taking their wives breast milk for the second twin to a hospital three hours drive away - we had it very easy. I heard the struggle many couples faced with young children and despised the fact that I had married a runner.

IVF was miraculous for me and had enhanced my life completely and, as far as I was concerned, was nothing in comparison to the years of infertility (it was those memories which still made me shudder) or the hardship of becoming a single mother of twins. It was an honest way of approaching a problem and I failed to see anything unnatural or wrong in it. I had firsthand experience of the power it had to enhance people's lives. Negative publicity was mean spirited; even the Pope once commented negatively on it, serving little purpose but making the loving parents and children involved feel rotten, especially the religious ones, and he was not in the best position to comment on the wellbeing of children right now...

    I tried to live and let live and accepted all religious or good paths as a decent road to travel as long as a person was nice about it. Just because I did one thing didn't mean it was right or the only way forward. I believed that we wouldn't have the ability to do such things, like resolve infertility or cure cancer, if it wasn't meant to be. Historically, people would have affairs to get the children they failed to get with their wives or husbands or accepted that empty feeling for life that some people cannot shake. How could my giving another couple a son they had desperately fought for be wrong? How could my beautiful, healthy and energetic twins be wrong? If they weren't meant to be then they simply would not be... They are a blessing. Jesus condemned adultery and God gave us the desperate desire to be parents. Nowhere in the bible is IVF criticised, only certain individuals claim such nonsense, and God or Mother Nature still has the last word in the outcome. I cannot see it as anything other than a gift and a blessing.

    IVF doesn't create life; eggs and sperm do. IVF was a medical intervention to help overcome whatever problem prevents the couple from achieving it alone and was not guaranteed. Should a woman who had acidic levels so high it destroyed her husband's sperm not seek support to have the family they dreamed of? Should trapped sperm not be helped to escape? These are people's hopes and dreams being smashed by often small obstacles that can be overcome with the right support.

    IVF was an extra battle and ordeal for a couple to face prior to the most life changing event in their lives – becoming parents.

I'd heard arguments against IVF that some career people actively choose to do IVF for convenience. There was nothing convenient about IVF. Years of trying to get pregnant destroyed my sex life if not my entire relationship and with hindsight, I wished I had done IVF two years earlier. My desire to get pregnant naturally now seemed irrelevant and a waste of time. You had no idea whether you had problems down the line awaiting you and time was not on your side. It was a practical and realistic choice and it was not a nice decision to have to make. I think it is also important to note the role of the anaesthetist's who seem to consistently make a good impression with couples with their positivity and conversational skills. They were fondly remembered by those of us who faced IVF and often don't get the appreciation they deserve. Thank you!

I could live a life without a man but a life without children would have been miserable for me. The thought of being stuck with James, without children, for the rest of my life was my idea of hell. Perhaps that says it all. I sometimes think of the boy I helped create, wondering if his parents were still together, and smiling at how much beauty had been created over the last few years, despite the tragedy of my marriage breakdown. I wondered if the couples divorcing who play games with their children, encourage them to take sides, drag them through the mud, would be the same if they hadn't had their children so easily? I felt horribly guilty for moaning about being tired or finding the twins too difficult because I had IVF. It was perfectly acceptable for a woman who conceived easily to moan but not for me. I always thought of those who had failed IVF and how ashamed I would be if they heard me. It was something I would always feel.

I was more my old self: calm and relaxed and able to handle conflict in the way I always used to - with humour or placidity. I was amazed at how much confrontation and aggression I attracted because of whatever my aura was sending out and how that had all changed with my attitude. It was as if aggressive and confrontational people seek out the weak but I was no longer seen as a target. I marvelled at how such people found you. I was grateful that the divorce was smooth, quick and amicable because it allowed me to move on and calm down far quicker than many other people I saw caught up in all the emotional baggage and bitterness of their divorce. It gave me a faster return to being a better person and therefore a better mother for the children.

Sadly, a few single mothers, including a sister, could not be friends with me because they were jealous of how amicable and easy my divorce was – and told me in no uncertain terms how easy I had it and didn't understand. I dared to suggest, tip-toeing on eggshells, that perhaps threatening to have his knees smashed in by a gypsy was not the best approach for an amicable divorce. A lot of women seemed to take no responsibility for the power they had on making things easy; they blamed it all on the man, it was never them - they simply didn't have a good man. I believed the woman had more power than they realised and no man, or woman, was at their best when it came to divorce but if one of you turned nasty it was essential the other one didn't. That was hard to achieve but I did it and it paid off dividends. Sadly, our relationship deteriorated after that, once James moved in with his new woman and insisted on dramatically changing the children's routine just as they started big school – I wouldn't allow it.

Nothing would take away the pain I have felt and continue to feel while a part of me is grieving over how it should have been. I have drank more than I should upon occasion and lost time depressed and miserable instead of being an energetic and loving mother. I've lowered myself by turning to drink or asking a neighbour to run to the shops for a packet of cigarettes – they wouldn't by the way, despite saying "if you ever need anything". I wonder if they would have gone if it had been calpol? I should have asked for calpol then, once they said yes, added the fags! I'm far from proud of myself but I resent how people judge you for drinking alone, when that is all you ever are, so should one go t-total at the most stressful time in your life? Or on the couple of occasions when I have gone out with neighbours and drank a lot, like everyone else, but married couples are "having a much deserved break from the kids" while I am being irresponsible. You never see married couples saying "you stay sober for the kids tonight" because they both have a drink. Why can't people say "that single mum works so hard, she's having a much deserved night off tonight, good for her!" It's all harsh negative judgement for the single parents of this world adding to our guilt and isolation.

Now my wine rack is full, I drink rarely and I keep a spare packet of cigarettes in case I ever break. There was a time when I felt like a fly in a pitcher plant and so desperately wanted to sink down into the nectar and die. Fortunately, I found strength and managed to crawl out and be the mother I should be. Only my love for the children gave me that. The twins were happy and they wouldn't be if James still lived here. He needed his own place and quiet time in order to be a decent father twice a month. He still comes once a week to do bath and bed with the kids but I don't like having him here or the way he treats me. I do it for the children. His father was no different; pay someone else to raise your children and just show off their photos to everyone – he kept his wife all to himself, and still does, whatever excuses are used. Father and son are very possessive men. I see her prison and lived it for a decade – that was long enough and perhaps I would have left if wanting children hadn't played such a big part? I loved being free. I understand that a lot of men struggle with the early years but where is the fight and maturity to do the right thing? We all struggle – it is no excuse to run.

I learn so much from the twins and I strive to be a good teacher in their life. I've no desire to domineer or control their path, shall open as many doors for them as I can, shall love and protect them along the way and learn as much as I can from their beautiful little characters. Painting their playhouse was something I'd rather not have done and I barely did it in the weekend that they were with their father. Hand painting their bedroom with African animals around a watering hole was far more fun. It's my way of keeping them with me even when they are away and helps pass the time. I still find it hard parting with them and sitting alone while they are away but I try to remain positive about it. I'm relieved he wants limited custody.

I finally get to the bottom of my health issues. The diary of symptoms I was keeping shows a pattern. From the day I ovulate until the day my period ends it's as if a switch is flicked and my entire body and mental state changes: my fingers and toes swell painfully into thick sausages; my stomach balloons as if I'm several months pregnant and it's rock hard; extreme fatigue – awaking more tired than when I go to bed; chronic back pain; reduced urination regardless of how much water I drink; blood with some bowel movement and sudden intermittent diarrhea when my kidneys fail. I gain and lose twelve pounds throughout each day with water retention. It feels as if, for this entire three week period in time, I am trying to drag my body through dense water. One day, upon picking the twins up from preschool, I dropped my foot on the clutch and that slight movement caused me to have a bowel movement, all watery, in the seat – with no warning. I told the GP I was far too young to be shitting myself and it's getting worse. I also explained that fudge knew there was something wrong by the way she kept sniffing my belly – that convinced me.

    Once kidney failure, or damage caused by the pre-eclampsia was ruled out, along with ovarian cancer, I am referred to a gynaecologist. The combination of endometriosis and severe PMS means my ovaries have to be shut down. I think the IVF drugs sent my ovaries into overtime. The gynaecologist who worked with my IVF said he suspected I had borderline polycystic ovaries since I created so many eggs during IVF. I am treated with zoladex, used for the treatment of cancer, a strong hormonal and mild chemotherapy injection I get each month to shut down my ovaries and force me into menopause along with HRT. Almost immediately I notice the difference and feel fantastic and my energy levels return to normal. I am given a new lease of life and it feels great. After having a break for two months from how I had been feeling I have a three day relapse whereby I return to that dark lethargic place and it is a shock to my system. Now I knew what it was like not to be like that, and to feel normal, I wonder how on earth I got through so many months of feeling that way. The feeling is horrible. It scares me. I don't know how I made it and how I managed to avoid suicide. I cry. I also cry every time I hear about a parent who kills their child and themselves on the news. Only my gratitude and love for the twins saw me through and I've learned how naturally kind and loving I am and could never hurt a child or an animal. I also know how pain, lack of sleep and illness makes me nasty so I need yoga daily, sufficient sleep and space when I'm not well. With babies this was not possible without support but now the children are older they will cuddle up and watch a movie with me while I sleep if I'm sick or have been up all night. It's much easier with older children.

The most wonderful part is that my chronic back problems vanished with the injections - endometriosis has been responsible for the chronic back pain since I was nineteen years old and I am overwhelmed with relief that is has gone. It isn't about how much endometriosis you have but where it is located but hormones seem to be the biggest cause. I cannot be cured but the menopause will be a good thing for me and hopefully shutting the ovaries down for a year will be enough to calm them and make life more bearable. If they treat the endometriosis the PMS will still be a problem and I'm too young for a full or part hysterectomy. I'm a rare and difficult case, I am told. It's lovely to feel good again and I wish I didn't feel bitter that it took so long to diagnose because of what James put me through – the GP naturally assumed it was depression and stress from the divorce. I try to overcome the bitterness that I had to have IVF because of him, it screwed up my body and he left me ill to raise the twins alone. I stay positive by thinking that it is hard to manage now, having to cut out caffeine, dairy and alcohol to make it better, but at least it isn't something I have to manage until the day I die – it will end with menopause. It is not until I feel normal that I realise just how bad I was. I cannot comprehend the power hormones have and what they have done to my body.

I get my hair highlighted and as the hairdresser dries my hair and I see how good it looks I burst out crying – I look and feel better than I have done in a long time. I'm reading a book to help me think more positively and not feel so sorry for myself. So much has happened to me over the last few years. I have gone from being a successful self-employed career woman, who earned more than my husband, to being a "society scrounger" and receiving a salary from the ex. I have no pride in my circumstances and not being able to earn my own way bothers me immensely. However, I am very lucky that the twins have been healthy and I've not had to do any hospital visits in the middle of the night – that would have been stressful – and we still have a nice house near a good school.

There are positives to divorcing early on: we weren't fighting and arguing in front of the children for years, I never had to move house and disrupt the children and I can be at home with them and ensure they feel loved and secure – even if no one else does – and this will be all they know. I'm in debt but simply cannot live on what is coming in despite my most frugal efforts and my attitude that I do not want the twins to go without during these precious years. If James or his family let the twins down I shall be there to pick up the pieces. I am their constant and strength in life. The twins understand that one parent isn't active in their lives but not why and we read them books and try to simplify this for them. I also write and draw our own books to help explain it. They understand he has left but not why.

I'm getting much better at the finances – my accountant did my finances and household finances was one of his jobs – taking on all *his* jobs has been a strange thing to come to terms with. I sell and buy a lot on ebay, carefully spread the money from breeding the dog, buy fish in bulk from a local farm, have organic fruit and vegetables delivered, they take healthy start vouchers, which forces me to make all my own food again. It's cheaper than visiting the supermarket, healthier and means I can go to bed earlier and feel better rested for the early start. I have to be extremely organised since I can't just pop out for anything, including medicine, and live far from shops.

I had a couple of lovely French students spend the summer and the twins third birthday with me and they were great company and help. I speak French and one was here for seven weeks – they were good friends to me and the children - I shall miss them both. One girl returned for another two weeks the following Easter which was wonderful. Fudge had another litter of puppies and the first one was hind feet first and it took a lot of nerve-racking effort to aid her with delivery. If this had happened with her first litter she would have needed to be rushed to the vets to have a caesarean – I could have lost her and the puppies. Fortunately, since this was her second litter we managed it and the nine puppies that followed were all head first and easy. It is a massive risk breeding a bitch when I have little money for reserves and fear losing the best friend I have. It could costs me hundreds if something went wrong.

I am a risk taker but it still worries me to death. I love the photo updates I've been receiving from the puppies I sold last year and they've all settled in well. It's such low earnings that it doesn't affect my Income Support for long. However, when I informed them that I had bred the dog they were rude, treated me like a criminal, made me post off every bank and visa statement I had and it stunned me. I wish I hadn't told them, their attitude made me think fraudulent behaviour was preferable because of the way they treated me – you wouldn't think I had rang up to confess to earning anything! All the puppies were reserved immediately: five during her pregnancy and the rest within a week of birth.

The charity that had the puppy last year, with no toes, is purchasing two as pets and I'm donating another to them. It goes amazingly well, ten puppies, five of each sex and I select a set of owners who seem the kindest people I have met in a long time who surprise me with the amount of respect they have for me. Most of them gave me or me and the twins a gift when they came to collect their puppy; toiletries, wine, champagne (which I drank as I cleaned the poop from the pens to store for another year) and I felt very moved. Both Fudge and I were much better this time around and it was easy in comparison to last year and all ten puppies passed their vet check. The Kennel Club came to visit and assess my house and said I had received lots of positive feedback.

Until I had the twins I was unaware of how I turned feelings of anger into self-destructive actions. I have learned so much from them already. There are books, TV and parenting courses to help improve my own knowledge to teach my children what I took so long to learn. I believe we cannot blame our parents for our mistakes and misfortunes once we have left home because we then have full responsibility for our own actions. I have grown so much from all of this and often think of boyfriends I have hurt and friends that I have sometimes let down without realising their acute pain and difficulties. I strive to be a better person from now on and I am doing a lot more for the community and isolated people. I have just applied for the twins school placement and shudder that the time is so near and I know how hard this is going to hit me. Regardless of the weather I shall wear sunglasses to hide the tears. I am not putting them in full time until they are five. It is a small and lovely school so I am tremendously glad we got to stay in the house.

Two years after he left James decides to tell me about his girlfriend, who just so happened to start working with him six months before he walked out on me but he claims they have only been together a short time. I don't believe him: she has met his parents, not something James would do in a young relationship and I was unfortunate enough to over-hear them talking negatively about me on the phone – they wouldn't talk in such a manner if it was a new relationship. I'm not jealous because I've known there was another woman from the start and just despise his weakness. The lying is insulting and only causes bad feeling. I still don't know if it was a succession of two women or the same one. He has passed all parental responsibility onto me and gives me extra money in the summer holidays towards activities rather than taking time off work to have them or takes just a couple of days off. I have no respect for him but try to remain amicable for the children. The twins and I have a wonderful bond and we are closer without James because I don't have to split my attention. Naturally, I am not happy about another woman being in my children's lives but then he won't be with another man – it's expected – we both have to come to terms with that. However, I have known there was someone else from the start, am used to the idea, feel no jealousy and know what she has. I only pity her as I relish my freedom from sulky-pants (as I now call him, only in my head, to make light of annoying situations).

We continue to go in and out of patches where we get on well enough or he is vile to me and I restrict him being here. It is hard to find a balance: I want him and the kids to spend time together but do not want them to grow up seeing me treated badly. He was at his worst when he moved in with his new girlfriend and his selfishness and new life took priority. Then, he resented what we cost him and wanted to alter the children's routine with no build up or time to allow them to adjust. I turn into the control freak at this point and start blackmailing legal custody rights to try and get James to do the right thing by the children – introduce change slowly. He hates me. I see it so clearly and although it hurts

I am used to it and bear it rather well nowadays. My only priority is to protect the children.

With hindsight, I can see how I was and how things I said may have upset people. Some people I knew were resentful or envious that I had twins, especially one of each sex, when they had a single baby. I made their complaints seem meagre, in their eyes, because I always had twice as much to deal with and a husband less – it made them feel uncomfortable when they complained about how tired or fed up they felt. I can see this now and I am glad to be rid of such people in my life because I desperately needed friendship. I have recently overheard many jealous comments from people, about their family or friends who have had twins, who don't realise I am a mother of twins, and am shocked at what they say. It's ironic more so because many mothers of twins have singleton envy, where they would love to have just one baby to bond and focus with, not to mention that you get left out when the twins have a close bond and play together for ages – often I try to play with them and they tell me to go away - it's a little sad really. Mothers of twins often feel a little left out but it is also nice that they have such a close bond.

I hate not having a career and miss working. My biggest resentment with James is how limited my options are as single mother – I can't have the career I used to have and attend meetings abroad without being able to leave them with their father – living in a rural area as a single mother makes long distance commuting impossible. I hate him for that. No one will hire me for anything less as they complain I am over-qualified. There are no local jobs – anything I earn would go on childcare and the kids loose me as well as their father. I will not be the sort of mother who has only an hour or two a day for her children. I asked James to sleep here two nights a week so I could work overnight in a nursing home – he refused – I'm utterly trapped. I want to work. There is no way I can work until they are both in full time school and my IT skills are long out of date.

I have had to sacrifice so much and nothing has changed for James; he has all his freedom, his career, a new girlfriend and sweeps in twice a month to have the children – but only for one night – he won't do two. His mother dropped him in it one day when I invited her round for tea, trying to make the effort again, when I explained that I wasn't stopping him from seeing them on a Friday. She told me that he and his girlfriend always go cycling after work on a Friday and wouldn't want to lose that. I couldn't believe it – father's for justice should lynch him!

I shall be on a much lower salary when they start school. I find that hard to swallow and feel the unfairness of it all. There are times I look at him and wonder why I ever loved him and how different life would have been with a loving and supportive husband. Then I only have to look at my children to realise he was, indeed, the best mistake I have ever made. He gave me these children. It is also limiting having to live with a disease, that I continue to fight daily, and the failed immune system with preschoolers means I am constantly sick. I catch and hold onto everything.

The medication helps immensely and eventually the normal pill suppresses my ovaries and I find myself with a normal body again – almost four years later. In many ways it is easier now the twins are older. Just being able to climb into their car seats alone is a massive help. In other ways it is harder because they are testing boundaries and absorb any energy my body manages to create. I am often unmotivated by the constant cleaning and laundry, especially in winter, and continue to feel overwhelmed. They rarely choke but when they do it is always together, which is frightening, but we always get through it. I lost Beth once at Peppa Pig world and it took a fifteen minute search to find her – she had stolen a teddy bear from the shop and ran off with it so I couldn't take it from her. It was the worst day of my life as terrifying thoughts of never seeing her again raced through my head. Day trips petrify me but I do them often and they both normally behave well. I'm determined to do normal things with them regardless of how stressful it is.

I would never wish to change what I have and have returned to a slimmer, calmer and happier self. Having worked long hours for international blue chip organisations I can honestly say I have never worked as hard as I have since the twins were born – going to work would be much easier. Staying at home is relentless, exhausting and often unchallenging. I am happy and privileged to have this time with them so I make the most of it and put one twin in preschool for a day each while I have quality time alone with the other twin. It allows me to teach them and enjoy them as individuals – they are quite different when separated. They talk me to death and make me laugh now and I love it. My second Christmas alone with them, aged three, was the happiest Christmas I have ever experienced. I ordered a precooked Turkey dinner and relished every moment of the holidays. It was such a relief.

They are both incredibly easy children unlike the cholic and lactose intolerant babies that never settled. I have had no terrible two's or tantrums and only minor phases to get through. They are calm, easy going and always go to bed easily. I don't know why they are so good but I know I have it easy. I feel privileged to be their mother. I adore watching their beaming smiles during Ballet, Gymnastics and Karate when they enjoy or achieve something. I shall always be grateful to IVF and James for giving me them no matter what. I'm also grateful that IVF allowed me to donate my eggs and give the remarkable gift of a child to another couple desperate for a family. It was a life changing and extraordinary experience. I have registered as a childminder, breed the dogs, and am home for the children. I have plenty of time for them, I'm organized and mostly have their school friends here so it works for us all. I have a lot of old friends in my life again now we can visit each other or meet at places with our children. I also have a lot of new friends and run a group for elderly people on Sundays which gives me a sense of pride in what I am doing in life again. Things are looking better.

The early years were certainly not what they should have been and I shall always feel sad for how it was. It is a sadness I can physically feel and makes me want to cry when I think about it. That time was taken away from me – my only opportunity to have young children and it was ruined in a way. It wasn't just James and him leaving me in emotional chaos at such a crucial time, it was the combination of what he did, my poor health, no local support and having two babies at the same time. I do regret my fling and cringe over it but I don't beat myself up – I was out of character. I started art at college one evening a week, which I love, and an MRI scan showed the injections had worked and everything was returning to normal and soon my body will have completely recovered – five years after birth! I get up at 05:30 and do yoga in peace and quiet before the day begins and enjoy that peaceful time to myself. My slipped disc is better now with yoga than it was ten years ago. Everything looks good. I no longer feel lonely. I finally like my own company and adore the company of the twins more now they're older. It's the little things like not being able to pop out for a run with the dogs when I like. It's frustrating. I use James as a free babysitter now – that is all he is to me.

  I shall probably always feel some sorrow in my heart for what the children have had to go through so early in life; how their father is so distant and not there for them as he should be and how I have been distracted with my own emotions and not there for them in the best way either. It is heartbreaking. However, I console myself with the fact that they are happy and balanced and we have a lot of fun together. We're close. I consider my parents who stayed married and how all five of us siblings are not happy with our childhood and continue to have no contact with our parents, or the one that still does, in an unhealthy manner. I know from personal experience that having two parents together is not always good either.

  There are some problems with the children and their emotional well-being but they will be OK. James refuses to talk with me or be involved in parenting in any way but he no longer listens to my advice on what will upset the children. It is hard managing a relationship like this. I do it alone and I do it well. I've battled with the frustration mothers have with finding work and how it's a catch-22 situation at every turn. I love having a sense of direction with being able to earn my own money again, albeit a very low paid option. For the first time in years I have a sense of purpose and pride in being independent. Once more I don't get the support I would like, in this instance from all neighbours, who don't see me trying to earn a living and just think of the noise in the house and garden. It seems I cannot win whatever I do. However, being the only child minder in the area does mean that everyone else is very supportive and our little village has no before or after school clubs so it's great for the village and many local parents are excited. I just hope this neighbour doesn't cause trouble and make the days unpleasant by complaining constantly. They complained about the noise of my own children, which surprised me since they have grown up children themselves. I feel awful and do not wish to spoil their quiet life – I just need to work.

My lack of freedom and mundane days are a small price to pay for two adorable children and all of my frustrations and pains will pass quickly. Since we split while they were so young I have hope of finding a nicer man in my life who will give me and them what we lack. However, another part of me loves being single and doesn't want a man in my life and it seems hard to find a man who doesn't need a lot of attention – perhaps I am biased?

Last night I put the twins to bed, in the usual way, and they snuggled under their duvets as I sang "Baby Mine" from Dumbo.

"Now it's sleep time," I said as I kissed and tucked them in. "Thank you for being good today, I had a wonderful time with you. Who is the best son in the whole wide world?"

"I am!" smiles Chris.

"That's right, and who is the best daughter in the whole wide world?"

"I am," shouts Beth gleefully.

I say a similar thing each night, perhaps ask them to be better behaved the next day, ensuring I always end with love and positivity - I'm very soft like that. They are both so good natured and easy going and go straight to sleep every night – they always have done unless they are sick. Tonight, for some unknown reason, I receive an extra response.

"Mummy?" Beth whispers.

"Yes?"

"Thank you for being a good mummy today too. I love you."

I choke up and smile. Beth talks like an adult sometimes and it's eerie, especially when I consider what sort of a mother I could have ended up being and it scares me.

"Mummy?"

"Yes, Chris?"

"I love you too much – right here," he says pointing to his heart and flashing me his teeth in that beautiful smile that lifts my heart every time. "You're a good mummy-son."

He doesn't quite understand the mother, son and daughter concept and it makes me smile through the tears in my eyes. I marvel at the beauty of these children and what little treasures they are. Staying at home with them was the best thing I could have done and I'm pleased, despite what I have lost on the career front. Having twins is lovely now because they do all their activities together. I feel smug watching other mum's running all over the place for their different aged children with mixed activities and breathe a sigh of relief that I don't have to juggle that. I give the twins a final kiss and squeeze when asked for an extra huggle and feel the warmth spread within. I have absolutely nothing to feel bad about anymore.

The end

Printed in Great Britain
by Amazon.co.uk, Ltd.,
Marston Gate.